Coagulation Disorders

Quality in Laboratory Diagnosis

D1376470

Diagnostic Standards of Care

MICHAEL LAPOSATA, MD, PHD
Series Editor

Coagulation Disorders
Quality in Laboratory Diagnosis
Michael Laposata, MD, PhD

Forthcoming in the Series
Clinical Microbiology

Diagnostic Standards of Care Series

Coagulation Disorders
Quality in Laboratory Diagnosis

Michael Laposata, MD, PhD
Edward and Nancy Fody Professor and
Executive Vice Chair of Pathology
Professor of Medicine
Vanderbilt University School of Medicine
Pathologist-in-Chief
Vanderbilt University Hospital
Nashville, Tennessee

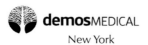
demosMEDICAL
New York

Acquisitions Editor: Richard Winters
Cover Design: Joe Tenerelli
Compositor: S4Carlisle Publishing Services
Printer: Hamilton Printing Company

Visit our website at www.demosmedpub.com

Medicine is an ever-changing science. Research and clinical experience are continually expanding our knowledge, in particular our understanding of proper treatment and drug therapy. The authors, editors, and publisher have made every effort to ensure that all information in this book is in accordance with the state of knowledge at the time of production of the book. Nevertheless, the authors, editors, and publisher are not responsible for errors or omissions or for any consequences from application of the information in this book and make no warranty, express or implied, with respect to the contents of the publication. Every reader should examine carefully the package inserts accompanying each drug and should carefully check whether the dosage schedules mentioned therein or the contraindications stated by the manufacturer differ from the statements made in this book. Such examination is particularly important with drugs that are either rarely used or have been newly released on the market.

Library of Congress Cataloging-in-Publication Data

Laposata, Michael.
 Coagulation disorders: quality in laboratory diagnosis / Michael Laposata.
    p. cm.—(Diagnostic standards of care)
 Includes bibliographical references and index.
 ISBN 978-1-933864-82-2 (alk. paper)
 1. Blood coagulation disorders—Diagnosis. 2. Diagnosis, Laboratory. I. Title. II. Series: Diagnostic standards of care.

 [DNLM: 1. Blood Coagulation Disorders—diagnosis. 2. Anticoagulants—therapeutic use. 3. Blood Coagulation—physiology. 4. Clinical Laboratory Techniques—methods. 5. Medical Errors—prevention & control. WH 322 L315c 2011]
 RC647.C55L37 2011
 616.1′57075—dc22

                                                                    2010021811

Special discounts on bulk quantities of Demos Medical Publishing books are available to corporations, professional associations, pharmaceutical companies, health care organizations, and other qualifying groups. For details, please contact:

Special Sales Department
Demos Medical Publishing
11 W. 42nd Street, 15th Floor
New York, NY 10036
Phone: 800–532–8663 or 212–683–0072
Fax: 212–941–7842
E-mail: rsantana@demosmedpub.com

Made in the United States of America
10 11 12 13 14   5 4 3 2 1

*To my wonderful brother, Sam, 12 years my senior,
who has loved, inspired, mentored, and emotionally
supported me for my entire life.*

Contents

Series Foreword

"Above all, do no harm." This frequently quoted admonition to healthcare providers is highly regarded, but despite that, there are few books, if any, that focus primarily on how to avoid harming patients by learning from the mistakes of others.

Would it not be of great benefit to patients if all health care providers were aware of the thrombotic consequences from heparin induced thrombocytopenia before a patient's leg is amputated? The clinically significant, often lethal, thrombotic events that occur in patients who develop heparin induced thrombocytopenia would be greatly diminished if all health care providers appropriately monitored platelet counts in patients being treated with intravenous unfractionated heparin.

It was a desire to learn from the mistakes of others that led to the concept for this series of books on diagnostic standards of care. As the test menu in the clinical laboratory has enlarged in size and complexity, errors in selection of tests and errors in the interpretation of test results have become commonplace, and these mistakes can result in poor patient outcomes. This series of books on diagnostic standards of care in coagulation, microbiology, transfusion medicine, hematology, clinical chemistry, immunology, and laboratory management are all organized in a similar fashion. Clinical errors, and accompanying cases to illustrate each error, are presented within all of the chapters in several discrete categories: errors in test selection, errors in result interpretation, other errors, and diagnostic controversies. Each chapter concludes with a summary list of the standards of care. The most common errors made by thousands of healthcare providers daily are the ones that have been selected for presentation in this series of books.

Practicing physicians ordering tests with which they are less familiar would benefit significantly by learning of the potential errors associated with ordering such tests and errors associated with interpreting an infrequently encountered test result. Medical trainees who are gaining clinical experience would benefit significantly by first understanding what not to do when it comes to ordering laboratory tests and interpreting test results from the clinical laboratory. Individuals working in the clinical laboratory would also benefit by learning of the common mistakes made by healthcare providers so that they are better able to provide helpful advice that would avert the damaging consequences of an error. Finally, laboratory managers and hospital administrators would benefit by having knowledge of test ordering mistakes to improve the efficiency of the clinical laboratory and avoid the cost of performing unnecessary tests.

If the errors described in this series of books could be greatly reduced, the savings to the healthcare system and the improvement in patient outcomes would be dramatic.

Michael Laposata, MD, PhD
Series Editor

Preface

The test menu in the clinical laboratory continues to dramatically increase in size and complexity. Over the past decade, reports that identify patient safety issues resulting from errors related to laboratory tests have started to emerge. Medical errors in this category have long been dismissed as being clinically inconsequential and financially irrelevant. The patient accounts in this book from a physician with more than 20 years of experience with coagulation disorders, as both a laboratory director and a clinical specialist, should dispel this conclusion.

There are many textbooks that describe an appropriate course of action to establish a diagnosis or to appropriately treat a patient. However, there are very few textbooks that focus on the errors to be avoided that compromise patient safety. This book on the standards of care in diagnostic coagulation describes commonly observed errors in test selection and result interpretation. I have directly witnessed many of the errors described in this book. Between 1995 and 2008, when I was a pathologist at the Massachusetts General Hospital and Harvard Medical School in Boston, I personally reviewed and created with trainees more than 20 000 individualized, expert-driven interpretations of complex evaluations from the special coagulation laboratory. In this role, I provided diagnostic information, upon review of both clinical and laboratory data, for virtually every coagulation evaluation that involved more than just the routine coagulation tests. I was exposed to many hundreds of errors in test selection and interpretation by physicians using the special coagulation laboratory at the Massachusetts General Hospital, which received samples from more than 70 hospitals. A major contributing factor for physicians' desire to use this laboratory was our provision of a patient-specific, expert-driven interpretation of the coagulation test results, which often educated physicians about laboratory test related errors. I shared a clinical practice for patients with disorders of hemostasis and thrombosis for more than 10 years in Boston, seeing patients directly as a specialist in the field. Some of the cases described in this book are related to problems reported to me by the patients in this practice who had encountered difficulty elsewhere. In some cases, the outcome was changed in this book to demonstrate an error that would have occurred if it had not been averted.

I have served as an expert witness or an expert consultant on a number of legal cases. This also exposed me to errors within my clinical expertise. In one case, to support the well-established recommendation to fully evaluate a persistently prolonged PT before neurosurgery, I was struck by the lack of authoritative references which I could have used as an expert on the witness stand. Unfortunately, in this case, "experts" were hired who testified that a prolonged PT before neurosurgery could simply be treated with fresh-frozen plasma without a determination of the cause of the prolonged PT! In two other cases, I was disappointed to learn that there was no standard of care in any textbook to indicate that a child with a subdural hematoma and a minor injury should be retested for von Willebrand disease if a normal set of test results was obtained in an initial analysis. In these legal cases, the children had undiagnosed von Willebrand disease, suffered minor injuries with serious bleeding episodes because of their bleeding disorders, and their fathers were accused of child abuse.

I would hope that all trainees and practicing physicians involved in the diagnosis of bleeding and thrombotic disorders would find it valuable to also learn what they should **not** do. Avoiding mistakes is a critical first step to optimizing patient outcome and maximizing patient safety.

Michael Laposata, MD, PhD

Acknowledgments

I would like to acknowledge Richard Winters, Executive Editor, Demos Medical Publishing, who patiently waited as this volume was enlarged by the addition of the cases, and who offered excellent advice from concept to completion of this work.

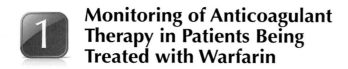

Monitoring of Anticoagulant Therapy in Patients Being Treated with Warfarin

OVERVIEW

Errors in anticoagulation therapy have become a major source of concern to hospital accrediting agencies. The simple error of not knowing about an elevated International Normalized Ratio (INR) value and therefore not taking an appropriate action is very common. Another common adverse outcome in warfarin-treated patients occurs from inappropriate decisions about dosing of warfarin, because many clinicians do not know the appropriate response to a supratherapeutic or subtherapeutic INR value. Such errors can result in catastrophic bleeding or thrombosis that is preventable. The laboratory can also contribute to error if it fails to use the correct formula for generation of the INR value.

TEST ORDERING MISTAKES

> Ordering the INR too soon after the initiation of warfarin therapy. The effect of warfarin occurs several days after the therapy is initiated. Checking the INR in the first 3 days of the administration of warfarin could lead to an inappropriate adjustment of the warfarin dose.

Case with Error

The doctor initiates warfarin therapy at 5 mg daily for a patient hospitalized with a pulmonary embolism. Before the patient is discharged the next day, the doctor checks the INR. The result is 1.3. The doctor concludes that this represents an insufficient warfarin dose and increases the dose to 7.5 mg daily before the patient leaves the hospital.

Explanation and Consequences

The anticoagulation action of warfarin is not fully present for several days after initiation of therapy. This is because warfarin reduces the synthesis of the active forms of factors II, VII, IX, and X, but it does not eliminate these coagulation factors from the circulation or inhibit their action. In this case, the patient now has an increased risk for bleeding from a warfarin overdose because a conclusion was made about the patient's response to warfarin before an appropriately timed assessment of the effect of warfarin was performed.

Not checking the INR value at least once per month. The maximum time interval for checking the INR value in a warfarin-treated patient is once per month, although there have been recent suggestions to lengthen this period in highly stable patients. Data now show the benefit of patients performing home testing for the INR. A meta-analysis revealed that patients who measure their own INR with a point of care device at home perform the INR 2 to 4 times more frequently than they would if they were managed by their physicians. Importantly, home-monitored patients with more frequent testing experience less bleeding and less thrombosis.

Case with Error

A patient has been receiving warfarin indefinitely since experiencing a second episode of venous thrombosis. Although the patient has been compliant with warfarin therapy, he has failed to have his INR checked for the past 4 months. He now presents with a third venous thrombosis, and his INR is found to be 1.3.

Explanation and Consequences

Many variables affect a patient's response to warfarin. Even in those patients whose INR value is within the therapeutic range 90% of the time, changes in diet, clinical condition, or medications can result in an increase or decrease in the warfarin effect. In this case, the patient experienced a diminished response to warfarin, and the consequences were a subtherapeutic INR and an associated thrombotic event.

▶ Determining the effect of warfarin reversal with vitamin K too soon. Many variables influence the time to reduction in INR with vitamin K therapy. For patients treated with oral vitamin K at a dose of 1 to 5 mg orally, the expectation is that a reduction in INR will occur within 24 hours; for those treated with vitamin K subcutaneously, the response is less predictable than it is for oral vitamin K, but in general, a reduction in INR should occur 6 to 12 hours sooner with subcutaneous administration than with oral administration; for intravenously delivered vitamin K, a reduction in the INR should be observed even sooner, typically within 12 hours.

Case with Error

A patient being treated with warfarin presents to the emergency room reporting hematuria with pink urine in the past 2 days. An INR value is obtained, and the result is 13. The patient is given 5 mg of vitamin K subcutaneously, and the warfarin is temporarily discontinued. The patient remains in the emergency room under observation. Four hours after receiving the subcutaneous injection of vitamin K, with all vital signs stable and no additional bleeding, the INR is checked again. The result is 10.9. The doctor concludes that a second subcutaneous injection of 5 mg vitamin K is required.

Explanation and Consequences

The subcutaneous injection of vitamin K will not take full effect within 4 hours. The action of vitamin K is to increase the synthesis of the active forms of factors II, VII, IX, and X, and the generation of a sufficient mass of these proteins in active form requires more than 4 hours.

RESULT INTERPRETATION MISTAKES

▶ Failing to review and act upon an INR value in a timely fashion. One of the most common mistakes occurs when the physician is unaware of an elevated INR value. This often happens when one physician is cross covering the patients of another physician and is unaware of the clinical status of the warfarin-treated patient for whom he or she has assumed temporary responsibility.

Case with Error

An orthopedic surgeon performs a hip replacement on a 75-year-old man. Postoperatively, the patient is given 5 mg warfarin daily for anti-coagulation. An INR is checked at the appropriate time, and the result is 9. The orthopedic surgeon who performed the hip replacement goes out of town, and her colleague is caring for her patients in her absence. The colleague fails to check the lab results for this gentleman, so no action is taken. The prolonged INR results in a major bleed at the site of the operation. The patient requires an emergency procedure and is given fresh frozen plasma to reverse the INR prolongation and stop the bleeding.

Explanation and Consequences

This is an extremely common circumstance and one that has been associated with much legal action over the years. INR values that are above the therapeutic range, especially in the period shortly after surgery, are extremely dangerous and must be appropriately treated in a timely fashion to minimize the risk of major bleeding.

▶Misunderstanding the clinical significance of an elevated INR value. Generally speaking, if there is a concern of serious bleeding in a warfarin-treated patient with a markedly elevated INR, usually above 9, fresh frozen plasma along with vitamin K needs to be administered to rapidly reverse the warfarin effect. Other approaches are evolving for replacement of factors II, VII, IX, and X. These involve the use of prothrombin complex concentrates containing these factors and the use of recombinant factor VIIa. Bleeding that does not appear to be life threatening can be treated with vitamin K, either subcutaneous or oral. Mildly elevated INR values can be treated by the temporary discontinuation of warfarin. In addition, an INR value significantly below the therapeutic range needs to be treated with an increase in the warfarin dose. In all cases, a thorough investigation for the cause of any supratherapeutic or subtherapeutic INR must be performed.

Case with Error

A patient receiving warfarin for atrial fibrillation presents to his physician for a regular checkup. As part of the evaluation, the doctor orders an INR. The result is 5.1. The patient is stable and shows no signs of bleeding. The doctor orders 2 units of fresh frozen plasma to be administered to the patient to normalize the elevated INR.

Explanation and Consequences

This is a case in which the patient is overtreated. For an INR elevation of 5.1 in the absence of bleeding for a patient with atrial fibrillation, discontinuing the warfarin for one or two nights and retesting the INR would be more appropriate. This patient has been unnecessarily exposed to the risks associated with receiving a blood product from a random donor.

▶Interpreting the INR value without qualification in the presence of interfering factors. One such example is for a patient receiving both argatroban and warfarin, with the goal of discontinuing the argatroban and continuing the warfarin long term. A therapeutic dose of argatroban will significantly elevate the INR in all patients. The INR value in the presence of argatroban should not be used to determine whether the patient is effectively anticoagulated with warfarin. Options include removing the argatroban for 2 to 3 hours and testing at that time with the INR or using a chromogenic factor X assay to monitor warfarin as this test does not suffer interference by argatroban.

Case with Error

A 68-year-old woman develops a pulmonary embolism and is treated with unfractionated heparin for 10 days. During the course of her hospital stay, her platelet count decreases, and she is found to have heparin-induced thrombocytopenia. The unfractionated heparin is discontinued, and she is placed on argatroban. Warfarin, at a dose of 5 mg daily, is added to the argatroban therapy, with plans to discontinue the intravenously delivered argatroban when warfarin produces its full anticoagulant effect. Her INR is measured during the time that she is receiving both warfarin and argatroban. The result is 17. The doctor concludes that the patient is highly sensitive to warfarin and that this is the primary cause for her markedly elevated INR value.

Explanation and Consequences

Argatroban strongly interferes with the INR, producing markedly elevated INR values. The INR is calculated from the PT. Because argatroban strongly inhibits thrombin in vivo and in vitro to produce its anticoagulation effect, it markedly prolongs the prothrombin time (PT) assay. The true INR cannot be determined in the presence of argatroban.

OTHER MISTAKES

▶ The failure of the laboratory to appropriately calculate the INR from the PT values generated from the patient samples. One of the major problems uncovered in clinical laboratories over the past decade is the incorrect calculation of the INR value. One cause for this incorrect calculation in some laboratories is that the value for the international sensitivity index (ISI) has been incorrectly assigned for the reagents in use to perform the PT assay from which the INR is calculated.

Case with Error

A clinical laboratory decides to purchase a new thromboplastin to perform the PT assay with an ISI value of 1. The current thromboplastin in use in the laboratory has an ISI value of 2. When the new thromboplastin arrives at the hospital, it is assumed that it is the desired product with an ISI value of 1. However, an error has led to the shipment of a lot of thromboplastin with an ISI value of 2. Without checking the new lot of thromboplastin to be certain that it is the desired product with an ISI of 1, the supervisor of the laboratory changes the formula for the INR calculation in the laboratory information system by inserting an ISI value of 1. Doctors in the hospital notice that there is a recent increase in the incidence of warfarin-associated hemorrhagic complications. After two patients suffer lethal intracranial bleeding, an investigation is performed. It reveals that the change in the ISI to a value of 1 in the laboratory information system, while the laboratory is using a thromboplastin with an ISI value of 2, has been producing INR results for the doctors that are falsely low. One patient with a target INR range of 2.5 to 3.5 is reported to have an INR of 2 when in reality it is 4. The doctor increases the warfarin dosage for this patient when informed that the INR is 2. The patient experiences a major bleed because in reality her INR is 4 at the time her warfarin dose is increased.

Explanation and Consequences

This case shows the dramatic consequences of incorrect anticoagulant dosing with warfarin. The doctors in this hospital had no way of knowing that the reagent in the laboratory used to perform the PT assay had been changed. Thus, they adjusted warfarin doses for patients as they had in the past to maintain their patients within the therapeutic INR range. By doing so, they unknowingly over-anticoagulated patients who were within or below the therapeutic range, which generated hemorrhagic complications.

CONTROVERSY

Using the INR as a replacement value for the PT in patients not receiving warfarin. The INR value is derived using data from patients who are being treated with warfarin. These patients have specific factor deficiencies (low levels of factors II, VII, IX, and X) that are a result of warfarin therapy. The clinical laboratory cannot easily know whether a sample for a PT test is from a warfarin-treated patient or a patient with liver disease, for example. Because there is a need to convert the PT value to an INR in the warfarin-treated patient, laboratory information systems typically convert all PT values into INR values. The clinicians then see values for both the PT and the INR for all patients for whom a PT test has been requested. The clinical use of the INR instead of the PT for non-warfarinized patients was originally discouraged. However, the INR appears to be an effective surrogate test for the PT, and now many clinicians follow the INR rather than the PT for patients with, for example, liver disease and disseminated intravascular coagulation (DIC).

> ▶ There is substantial controversy about the merits of phar-
> macogenomic testing to assess for warfarin sensitivity.
> The FDA supports such testing, but the logistical challenge is
> very high to determine the status of CYP2C9 (3*/3* genotype
> patients should be treated with a lower warfarin dose) and vita-
> min K epoxide reductase (VKORC1, the AA genotype patients
> benefit from a lower warfarin dose) within the first few days of
> warfarin therapy and permit early dose adjustment. There is
> now significant data to show that pharmacogenomic testing for
> warfarin sensitivity shortens the time to stable dosing and
> increases the time that patients receiving warfarin are within the
> therapeutic range.

STANDARDS OF CARE

▦ Patients receiving warfarin must be monitored using the INR.
Warfarin dose adjustment should not occur until the patient has
received two to three doses of warfarin and monitoring should
occur at least once per month.

▦ Subtherapeutic and supratherapeutic INR values must be acted
upon in a timely fashion to minimize the risk of bleeding or thrombosis. Values that are substantially outside the therapeutic range
require immediate attention to prevent a potentially lethal outcome.

▦ When the INR does not reflect the effect of warfarin alone, but is
confounded by other variables, warfarin dose adjustment must take
into account such confounders.

▦ The laboratory must correctly calculate the INR from the PT value
of the patient.

2 Monitoring of Anticoagulant Therapy in Patients Being Treated with Unfractionated Heparin

OVERVIEW

Patients receiving unfractionated heparin are most commonly monitored using the partial thromboplastin time (PTT) assay. However, many clinical laboratories monitoring heparin-treated patients are now using an assay for anti-factor Xa. There is substantial variability in patient response to unfractionated heparin therapy. In addition, the laboratory reagent used in the performance of the PTT shows lot-to-lot variability, and this can introduce substantial analytical variability in the PTT. Thus, the biological and the analytical variability associated with heparin treatment make it difficult to continuously maintain a patient within the therapeutic PTT range. As with all anticoagulants, errors surrounding anticoagulation therapy have become highly visible because they can result in catastrophic bleeding or thrombosis, and they are often preventable. Another major complication associated with heparin therapy is the development of heparin-induced thrombocytopenia (HIT) with thrombosis (see Chapter 6 on HIT). Monitoring the platelet count in a hospitalized patient on intravenous unfractionated heparin therapy is essential to reduce the incidence of this potentially lethal thrombotic condition by discontinuing heparin therapy and introducing an anticoagulant unrelated to heparin.

TEST ORDERING MISTAKES

▶ Not ordering a platelet count at least every third day while a patient is in the hospital receiving unfractionated heparin, as an assessment for HIT.

Case with Error

A 78-year-old man is admitted to the hospital for consideration of a coronary artery bypass graft procedure. Upon admission, his platelet count is 248 000 per microliter. He is placed on intravenous heparin for therapeutic anticoagulation for 10 days, during which time his platelet count is not checked. On the 11th hospital day, a platelet count is performed and found to be 48 000 per microliter. Without further evaluation of the cause of the thrombocytopenia, a decision is made to proceed with the operation. This operation involves a cardiopulmonary bypass pump, which is primed with large amounts of unfractionated heparin. Three hours before surgery, the patient receives 12 units of platelets. Within 2 days of the procedure, the patient suffers massive thrombosis resulting in amputation of both legs. A test for antibodies to the heparin–platelet factor 4 complex associated with HIT is markedly positive.

Explanation and Consequences

It is likely that this patient experienced a declining platelet count sometime between admission and the 11th hospital day as he developed HIT. Patients with this disorder, who experience thrombocytopenia, are at high risk of developing the thrombotic complications associated with this condition. Because no platelet counts were performed for 10 days, the doctors were not aware of this thrombotic risk, which could have led to prevention of his thrombosis. Two cardinal errors were made in this case for a patient with HIT—continued exposure to heparin and the administration of platelet concentrates.

Requesting an anti-factor Xa assay to monitor the effect of unfractionated heparin, but not indicating to the laboratory that the test is assessing the effect of unfractionated heparin. Low molecular weight heparin is also monitored by an anti-factor Xa assay. The laboratory uses unfractionated heparin to calibrate the assay when the anticoagulant effect of unfractionated heparin is being assessed; and it uses low molecular weight heparin when the anticoagulant effect of low molecular weight heparin is being assessed. The laboratory must know, therefore, whether the test request is for the assessment of anticoagulation with unfractionated heparin or low molecular weight heparin.

Case with Error

A 38-year-old woman being treated with unfractionated heparin for a deep vein thrombosis is evaluated by her doctor with an anti-factor Xa assay. The laboratory presumes that the patient is being treated with low molecular weight heparin and produces a test result for anti-factor Xa from an assay using low molecular weight heparin standards to calibrate the assay. The test result is incorrect. This is not known to the doctor who is unaware that the anti-factor Xa assay for unfractionated heparin is performed differently from the anti-factor Xa test for low molecular weight heparin.

Explanation and Consequences

The doctor receives a result that is not in the therapeutic range for anti-factor Xa. An inappropriate adjustment of unfractionated heparin dosing occurs. If an anti-factor Xa assay is calibrated with low molecular weight heparin standards, and the anti-factor Xa for low molecular weight heparin is 0.6, the anti-factor Xa for unfractionated heparin calibrated as such is 1.0. It should be noted that different low molecular weight heparin preparations, for example, Lovenox and Fragmin, can be used interchangeably as calibrators for an anti-factor Xa assay involving measurement of a low molecular weight heparin concentration.

RESULT INTERPRETATION MISTAKES

▶ Failing to review and act upon a supratherapeutic or sub-therapeutic PTT value in a patient being treated with unfractionated heparin value in a timely fashion. The consequences for a patient requiring anticoagulation with unfractionated heparin whose PTT is not in the therapeutic range are bleeding (for PTT values above the therapeutic range) and thrombosis (for PTT values below the therapeutic range). The bleeding or thrombotic events can range from mild to lethal, and for that reason, maintenance of the heparin-treated patient within the therapeutic PTT range greatly improves patient outcome.

Case with Error

A patient with a history of duodenal ulcers being treated with unfractionated heparin for a pulmonary embolism develops a PTT value of greater than 150 seconds. The doctor receives notification of a panic value for the PTT. No action is taken over the next 3 hours, and the patient suffers a catastrophic gastrointestinal hemorrhage.

Explanation and Consequences

Laboratory values that are outside the target range, reflecting inappropriate anticoagulation, require immediate attention to avoid serious adverse outcomes, as illustrated in this case.

> ▶ Failing to pursue a diagnosis of HIT upon observing a
> decline in the platelet count to 50% or less of the baseline
> platelet count, in a patient exposed to unfractionated heparin or
> low molecular weight heparin by any route and at any dose,
> particularly in the absence of an alternative explanation for the
> decrease in platelets.

Case with Error

A patient's platelet count decreases from 300 000 per microliter to
100 000 per microliter within 1 week after a single subcutaneous
injection of 5000 units of unfractionated heparin. No further exposure
to heparin occurs during the next 5 days in the hospital. A diagnosis of
HIT was not considered because the doctor concluded that only intravenously administered, full-dose unfractionated heparin could lead to
the development of HIT.

Explanation and Consequences

This missed diagnosis of HIT resulted in arterial thrombosis and loss
of the patient's left foot. The single subcutaneous injection of unfractionated heparin as a prophylaxis against thrombosis is an adequate
stimulus to produce HIT with thrombotic complications.

▶ Concluding that the PTT is within the therapeutic range in a patient receiving heparin, who also has a lupus anticoagulant or other condition associated with a prolonged PTT, such as factor XII deficiency. Using the lupus anticoagulant as an example, the lupus anticoagulant can prolong the PTT. However, this prolongation is not reflective of an anticoagulation effect. If a patient with a lupus anticoagulant develops thrombosis and requires treatment with heparin, and the PTT is already elevated above the upper limit of normal before heparin treatment, the patient may receive an inadequate amount of heparin if the physician uses the standard PTT therapeutic range to adjust heparin dosing. In such cases, the PTT cannot be used to assess the effectiveness of anticoagulation with heparin. The anti-factor Xa assay for unfractionated heparin must be used in these cases. Providing a thrombotic patient with an inadequate dose of unfractionated heparin can result in clinically significant thrombosis.

Case with Error

A 28-year-old woman with autoimmune disease develops a deep vein thrombosis. A laboratory evaluation from a blood sample collected before the initiation of any anticoagulant therapy reveals the presence of a prolonged PTT of 55 seconds and a positive test for the lupus anticoagulant. The doctor treats the deep vein thrombosis with unfractionated heparin with a target range of 60 to 90 seconds. The maintenance dose for this target range is found to be unusually low at 5 mg/kg/h. While on this heparin dose, the patient develops a massive pulmonary embolism and is transferred to the intensive care unit.

Explanation and Consequences

When the PTT is elevated before the initiation of heparin therapy, a PTT therapeutic range cannot be used. In this case, the PTT therapeutic range of 60 to 90 seconds was used when the PTT was already elevated to 55 seconds by the lupus anticoagulant, and therefore, an inadequate amount of heparin was provided to the patient. The under-dosing of heparin permitted the development of the massive pulmonary embolism. In such cases, unfractionated heparin must be monitored with an assay for anti-factor Xa instead of the PTT.

> Confusing the therapeutic range in the anti-factor Xa assay for unfractionated heparin (0.3–0.7 U/mL) with that of the therapeutic range for low molecular weight heparin (0.5–1.0 U/mL).

Case with Error

A patient being treated with unfractionated heparin has an anti-factor Xa value of 1.0 U/mL. The doctor is most familiar with the therapeutic range for anti-factor Xa in patients being treated with low molecular weight heparin, which is 0.5 to 1.0 U/mL. It is presumed by the doctor that the value of 1.0 is at the upper end of the therapeutic range, when in fact it is well above the upper limit of the therapeutic anti-factor Xa range for unfractionated heparin. The patient develops spontaneous bruising.

Explanation and Consequences

Most patients monitored with anti-factor Xa levels are those receiving low molecular weight heparin. Occasionally, however, patients being treated with unfractionated heparin require monitoring with anti-factor Xa levels instead of the PTT. The over-anticoagulation in this case resulted in the spontaneous bruising, and it resolved when the dosage of unfractionated heparin was reduced and the patient was maintained within the anti-factor Xa target range of 0.3 to 0.7 U/mL.

▶ Expecting a therapeutic PTT or a therapeutic anti-factor Xa level after treatment with prophylactic unfractionated heparin doses, commonly 5000 units 2 or 3 times per day. Prophylactic doses do not produce therapeutic levels unless there is a confounding variable also prolonging the PTT.

Case with Error

A patient with pneumonia receives 5000 units of unfractionated heparin 3 times per day as a prophylactic measure against venous thrombosis. The doctor checks the PTT value for this patient, and the result shows that the value is not elevated. The doctor presumes that this represents a laboratory error and for that reason retests the patient with another PTT test. The result of this second test is also completely normal at 32 seconds.

Explanation and Consequences

Prophylactic doses of unfractionated heparin often do not prolong the PTT or elevate it only slightly. In this case, the second test was unnecessary.

OTHER MISTAKES

▶ Samples from heparinized patients in whole blood will have a declining PTT value as they remain in whole blood for several hours before the analysis. Activation of even a small percentage of the platelets in whole blood results in the release of a substance from the activated platelets that neutralizes heparin. The clinical impact of this preanalytical error is that the patient may have a therapeutic PTT in vivo that is inappropriately observed to be subtherapeutic, or a supratherapeutic PTT that is incorrectly perceived as therapeutic. The clinical impact of either of the situations is incorrect heparin dosing of the patient. A standard recommendation is that a whole-blood specimen is processed to separate blood cells from plasma within 4 hours of sample collection.

Case with Error

A 58-year-old diabetic patient is receiving heparin therapy. After a bolus of unfractionated heparin at a standard loading dose, the patient is placed on a maintenance dose of intravenous unfractionated heparin to maintain a target PTT range of 60 to 90 seconds. For 3 days, the PTT values are within this therapeutic range with no change in heparin dose. On the fourth day, a PTT is performed, and the result is 41 seconds, which is only slightly elevated and markedly different from recent PTT values. An investigation reveals that the sample remained in the laboratory at room temperature before analysis for 6 hours.

Explanation and Consequences

This is a particularly common occurrence when samples are transported with a delay in the analysis. The transportation time alone prolongs the interval between blood collection and performance of the PTT. Samples can be transported and still be suitable for performance of a PTT for heparin monitoring if they are first centrifuged, and the plasma is removed to separate it from platelets, which release substances that can neutralize heparin in the plasma. The danger to the patient in such cases is that the PTT is falsely low, and the doctor may respond by increasing the dose of heparin and over-anticoagulate the patient.

CONTROVERSY

There is substantial controversy for patients receiving unfractionated heparin on whether the use of the anti-factor Xa assay for monitoring unfractionated heparin is more reflective of bleeding and thrombotic risk than the PTT. The assay for anti-factor Xa in the clinical laboratory is much more expensive than the PTT, and it is also more complex and therefore requires more sophisticated instrumentation than the PTT. These limitations notwithstanding, many clinical laboratories have instituted heparin monitoring with anti-factor Xa assays.

STANDARDS OF CARE

- Patients receiving unfractionated heparin must be monitored for bleeding and thrombotic complications using either a therapeutic PTT range or a therapeutic anti-factor Xa range for unfractionated heparin. Supratherapeutic and subtherapeutic PTT or anti-factor Xa values must be acted upon in a timely fashion to minimize the risk of bleeding or thrombosis.
- Patients receiving unfractionated heparin, especially those in the hospital, should be monitored for the development of HIT with platelet counts at least every third day.

▓ Patients who have a prolonged PTT before the initiation of heparin therapy cannot be monitored with the PTT assay to determine heparin dosing. An anti-factor Xa assay must be used in these cases, with careful attention to use the therapeutic range associated with unfractionated heparin and not low molecular weight heparin.

▓ Specimens to be evaluated with a PTT assay to assess the effect of heparin anticoagulation must be processed to separate plasma from blood cells within 4 hours of collection to avoid preanalytical neutralization of heparin in the specimen.

3

Monitoring of Anticoagulant Therapy in Patients Being Treated with Low Molecular Weight Heparin

OVERVIEW

Unlike unfractionated heparin, the biological and analytical variability associated with low molecular weight heparin treatment is highly reproducible. For this reason, it is unnecessary to monitor the anticoagulation effect of low molecular weight heparin in most patients. For those patients who do need monitoring (see section Result Interpretation Mistakes for indications), the appropriate test is the anti-factor Xa assay. As with all anticoagulants, errors surrounding anticoagulation therapy have become highly visible, because such errors can result in catastrophic bleeding or thrombosis, and they are often preventable. Although it is less common in patients receiving low molecular weight heparin than unfractionated heparin, a serious complication associated with low molecular weight heparin therapy is the development of heparin-induced thrombocytopenia with thrombosis (see Chapter 6 on heparin-induced thrombocytopenia). The platelet count in patients receiving low molecular weight heparin, for several compelling reasons described in this chapter, is monitored less often than it is for hospitalized patients receiving unfractionated heparin.

TEST ORDERING MISTAKES

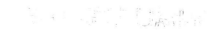Ordering a PTT assay to monitor anticoagulation with low molecular weight heparin instead of the anti-factor Xa assay. Low molecular weight heparin treatment, even at therapeutic doses, results in only a mild prolongation of the PTT in most cases.

Case with Error

A patient is treated for pulmonary embolism with the low molecular weight heparin Lovenox at 1 mg/kg 2 times per day. The doctor orders a PTT to monitor the anticoagulant effect of low molecular weight heparin. The PTT is normal. The doctor increases the dose of Lovenox to 1.5 mg/kg 2 times per day. When the hematocrit is found to be decreasing in the presence of this higher dose of low molecular weight heparin, an investigation is performed, and the doctor is informed that the PTT is not elevated to any appreciable extent even with therapeutic doses of low molecular weight heparin in most patients.

Explanation and Consequences

When low molecular weight heparin was first introduced, many doctors presumed that the PTT would be used to monitor this drug because the PTT is used to monitor unfractionated heparin. Though most physicians now understand that the PTT is not used to monitor the anticoagulant effect of low molecular weight heparin, many physicians remain unfamiliar with the anti-factor Xa assay, particularly how and when it is used to monitor the anticoagulant effect of low molecular weight heparin.

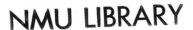

Requesting an anti-factor Xa assay to monitor the effect of low molecular weight heparin, but not indicating to the laboratory that the test is assessing the effect of low molecular weight heparin. Unfractionated heparin is also monitored by an anti-factor Xa assay. The laboratory uses low molecular weight heparin to calibrate the assay when the anticoagulant effect of low molecular weight heparin is being assessed, and it uses unfractionated heparin when the anticoagulant effect of unfractionated heparin is being assessed. The laboratory must know, therefore, whether the test request is assessing anticoagulation with low molecular weight heparin or unfractionated heparin.

Case with Error

See the second case in Chapter 2 on monitoring unfractionated heparin therapy for an illustrative case in which the incorrect calibration curve is used.

RESULT INTERPRETATION MISTAKES

▶Failing to review and act upon a supratherapeutic or sub-therapeutic anti-factor Xa value in a patient being treated with low molecular weight heparin in a timely fashion. This applies only to patients who have a requirement for being monitored while receiving low molecular weight heparin. The majority of patients receiving low molecular weight heparin do not require monitoring with any assay to assess the extent of anticoagulation. Indications for monitoring include renal impairment; elevated body mass index; low body mass index; pregnancy; infancy, especially in the neonatal period; and long-term anticoagulation with low molecular weight heparin. The consequences for patients requiring anticoagulation with low molecular weight heparin whose anti-factor Xa is not in the therapeutic range are bleeding (for anti-factor Xa values above the therapeutic range) and thrombosis (for anti-factor Xa values below the therapeutic range). As with all anticoagulants, the bleeding or thrombotic events can range from mild to lethal, and for this reason maintenance of the patient treated with low molecular weight heparin within the therapeutic anti-factor Xa range is absolutely essential.

Case with Error

A 25-year-old woman with a body mass index of 17 is treated with low molecular weight heparin for deep vein thrombosis. The result for the anti-factor Xa assay, ordered in this case because of the low body mass index, is 1.4 U/mL. The doctor rapidly responds to this value by decreasing the dose of low molecular weight heparin for the next subcutaneous injection. No bleeding complications occur.

Explanation and Consequences

This is the expected outcome when there is a timely response to an elevated value for anti-factor Xa in a patient being treated with low molecular weight heparin. Complications were avoided because of prompt dose adjustment. In addition, the doctor understood that the low body mass index was among several indications that should prompt the monitoring of low molecular weight heparin.

> Failing to pursue a diagnosis of heparin-induced thrombo-cytopenia upon a decline in the platelet count to 50% or less of the baseline platelet count in a patient exposed to low molecular weight heparin by any route at any dose, in the absence of an alternative explanation for the decrease in platelets. Although unfractionated heparin is more frequently associated with heparin-induced thrombocytopenia, exposure to low molecular weight heparin alone can produce heparin-induced thrombocytopenia.

Case with Error Averted

A patient in a rehabilitation hospital being treated with low molecular weight heparin as prophylaxis against thrombosis after knee replacement surgery develops a platelet count that declines to an extent and at a rate consistent with heparin-induced thrombocytopenia. The patient is found to have antibodies to the heparin–platelet factor 4 complex. The low molecular weight heparin is discontinued, and prophylaxis against thrombosis is initiated with argatroban. The platelet count returns over the next several days to normal. The patient does not develop thrombotic complications.

Explanation and Consequences

It may be difficult to monitor platelet counts in patients being treated with low molecular weight heparin because they are often at home when they are taking the medication. In this case, the patient was in a rehabilitation hospital, and in that setting, assessment of the platelet count was not difficult. The identification of the heparin-induced thrombocytopenia in this patient may have prevented a significant thrombotic event.

> Confusing the therapeutic range in the anti-factor Xa assay for low molecular weight heparin (0.5–1.0 U/mL) with that of the unfractionated heparin (0.3–0.7 U/mL).

Case with Error

A patient being treated with low molecular weight heparin has an anti-factor Xa value of 0.3 U/mL. The doctor confuses the therapeutic range for unfractionated heparin, which is 0.3 to 0.7 U/mL, with the therapeutic range for low molecular weight heparin, which is 0.5 to 1.0 U/mL. He mistakenly concludes that this value is within the therapeutic range when, in fact, it is subtherapeutic for a patient on low molecular weight heparin. A deep vein thrombosis develops in the patient, and this leads to further education of the doctor and an increase in the dose of low molecular weight heparin provided to the patient to achieve a value within the anti-factor Xa target range of 0.5 to 1.0 U/mL.

> Expecting a therapeutic anti-factor Xa level after treatment with prophylactic low molecular weight heparin doses. Treatment with prophylactic doses of low molecular weight heparin produces anti-factor Xa levels that are well below the therapeutic range.

Case with Error

A 42-year-old patient recovering from abdominal surgery is receiving a prophylactic dose of the low molecular weight heparin Lovenox at 40 mg daily by subcutaneous injection. The doctor orders an assay for anti-factor Xa to monitor the anticoagulant effect of the low molecular weight heparin. The value obtained is 0.1 U/mL, which is well below the therapeutic range for low molecular weight heparin. The doctor questions the laboratory on why the value is subtherapeutic when it is the standard recommended dose for prophylaxis against venous thrombosis.

Explanation and Consequences

Prophylactic doses of low molecular weight heparin do not increase the anti-factor Xa level to the therapeutic range, much like prophylactic doses of unfractionated heparin do not prolong the PTT into the PTT therapeutic range.

OTHER MISTAKES

▶ Not collecting a blood sample for anti-factor Xa monitoring of the patient treated with low molecular weight heparin at 4 hours after subcutaneous administration of the low molecular weight heparin. The therapeutic effect of low molecular weight heparin is assessed at 4 hours postinjection. Values before and after 4 hours (within a window of about 15–30 minutes) will be different from those obtained at 4 hours, and the misleading laboratory result could lead to inappropriate adjustment of the low molecular weight heparin dose.

Case with Error

A hospitalized patient being treated with a therapeutic dose of low molecular weight heparin for a pulmonary embolism is being monitored with an assay for anti-factor Xa. The sample collected for monitoring is obtained 6 hours after the most recent subcutaneous injection of low molecular weight heparin. The value for anti-factor Xa is 0.2 U/mL, which is well below the therapeutic range of 0.5 to 1.0 U/mL. The doctor interprets this result as inadequate dosing of low molecular weight heparin and increases the amount of low molecular weight heparin for subcutaneous injection. Two days after initiation of the higher dose, the patient develops an episode of spontaneous epistaxis and significant hematomas when blood samples are collected.

Explanation and Consequences

Samples collected for monitoring low molecular weight heparin must be collected very close to 4 hours after the most recent subcutaneous injection. It is the value for the anti-factor Xa assay at this time that is most predictive of both antithrombotic efficacy and bleeding risk. Samples collected well after 4 hours, as in this case, typically show lower anti-factor Xa levels than expected because more time has elapsed since the most recent administration of the anticoagulant. This case is an example of one in which a dosing error occurred because of a mistake in the timing of sample collection.

> ▶ Whole-blood samples from patients treated with low molecular weight heparin will show a declining anti-factor Xa value as the time between sample collection and analysis is increased. For this reason, whole-blood samples must be centrifuged to separate the blood cells from the plasma. Activation of even a small percentage of the platelets in whole blood results in the release of platelet factor 4 from the activated platelets, which neutralizes heparin and low molecular weight heparin. The clinical impact of this preanalytical error is that the patient may have a therapeutic anti-factor Xa in vivo that is inappropriately deemed subtherapeutic, or have a true supratherapeutic anti-factor Xa that is incorrectly perceived as therapeutic. The clinical impact of either of the situations is incorrect dosing of the patient with low molecular weight heparin. As with unfractionated heparin, a standard recommendation is that a whole-blood specimen is processed to separate blood cells from plasma within 4 hours of sample collection.

Case with Error Averted

A 42-year-old obese woman is receiving low molecular weight heparin therapy for deep vein thrombosis. Because of her elevated body mass index, her low molecular weight heparin is being monitored with an assay for anti-factor Xa. Although her first two values show results in the middle of the therapeutic range, her most recent value is extremely sub-therapeutic. An investigation reveals that the blood sample with the low value remained as whole blood at room temperature for 8 hours before analysis. Because the anti-factor Xa value appeared spurious to the doctor, no change in low molecular weight heparin dosing was made.

Explanation and Consequences

As with unfractionated heparin, low molecular weight heparin can also be neutralized by platelet factor 4, which is released from platelets in samples of whole blood before analysis. This results in a falsely low value for anti-factor Xa and increases the possibility that the doctor may respond by increasing the dose of low molecular weight heparin, to the detriment of the patient.

CONTROVERSY

▶ Not ordering a platelet count at least every third day for the patient receiving low molecular weight heparin, at least while a patient is in the hospital, and not beginning platelet count checks on the fourth day following initial heparin exposure, as an assessment for heparin-induced thrombocytopenia. Although monitoring the platelet count for patients receiving unfractionated heparin in the hospital to assess for heparin-induced thrombocytopenia is well accepted, monitoring the platelet count for patients receiving low molecular weight heparin is controversial. This is because low molecular weight heparin is often given for treatment of outpatients, and it is more difficult to test outpatients than inpatients, especially on a regular basis, for the platelet count. In addition, the risk for development of heparin-induced thrombocytopenia after exposure to low molecular weight heparin is less than it is for unfractionated heparin. Finally, there is appropriate widespread use of prophylactic anticoagulation of hospitalized patients with low molecular weight heparin to prevent thrombosis. Monitoring of platelet counts in this population would require platelet counts of a large number of hospitalized patients. Generally speaking, many experts would consider it advisable to monitor the platelet count at some point during hospitalization for a patient receiving therapeutic doses of low molecular weight heparin.

STANDARDS OF CARE

▨ Patients receiving low molecular weight heparin who must be monitored for bleeding and thrombotic complications are evaluated using an anti-factor Xa assay with a therapeutic range for low molecular weight heparin of 0.5 to 1.0 U/mL.

▨ Subtherapeutic and supratherapeutic anti-factor Xa values must be acted upon in a timely fashion to minimize the risk of bleeding or thrombosis. Values that are substantially outside the therapeutic range require immediate attention to prevent a potentially lethal outcome.

▦ Although it is controversial, it is a safe practice for patients receiving low molecular weight heparin, especially those in the hospital and who are receiving treatment doses of low molecular weight heparin, to be monitored for the development of heparin-induced thrombocytopenia with platelet counts at some point.

▦ For monitoring the effect of low molecular weight heparin with an anti-factor Xa assay, samples must be collected 4 hours after the subcutaneous injection of low molecular weight heparin. Dosing of low molecular weight heparin is based on the value collected at this time, and dose adjustment based on results of samples collected more than 30 minutes before or after 4 hours may be incorrect.

▦ Whole-blood specimens to be evaluated with an anti-factor Xa assay to assess the effect of low molecular weight heparin anticoagulation must be processed to separate plasma from blood cells within 4 hours of collection to avoid the preanalytical neutralization of low molecular weight heparin in the specimen.

Monitoring of Anticoagulant Therapy in Patients Being Treated with Fondaparinux

OVERVIEW

Fondaparinux is a pentasaccharide that is chemically synthesized, unlike unfractionated heparin and its derivative low molecular weight heparin, which are derived from pig intestine. Its pharmacokinetics is so reproducible in nearly all patients with adequate renal function that it is rarely necessary to monitor its anticoagulation effect. The reproducibility of the pharmacologic effect is comparable or better than that found for low molecular weight heparin. For those patients who do require monitoring, the appropriate test is the anti-factor Xa assay. Patients who have moderate to severe renal impairment must not receive this anticoagulant, as it is cleared exclusively by the kidney. Monitoring may be highly informative in a patient with renal disease who inappropriately received fondaparinux and begins to bleed.

Importantly, fondaparinux has no well-established reversibility agent. Protamine sulfate can be used to neutralize unfractionated heparin and much of the activity of low molecular weight heparin, but it does not neutralize fondaparinux. In addition, the half-life for fondaparinux is on the order of 20 hours, unlike low molecular weight heparin with a half-life of about 5 hours and unfractionated heparin with a half-life of approximately 1 hour. It is extremely rare to identify a fondaparinux-treated patient who has a clinically significant complication of HIT (see Chapter 6 on HIT). Monitoring the platelet count in patients receiving fondaparinux, therefore, is not indicated.

TEST ORDERING MISTAKES

 Failing to measure the creatinine or other assessment of renal function before administering fondaparinux.

Case with Error

A 68-year-old woman receives a therapeutic dose of fondaparinux for a spontaneous deep vein thrombosis. Although she receives the appropriate weight-based dose, she develops gastrointestinal bleeding. An assessment of her renal function, after she has received a subcutaneous injection of fondaparinux, shows a moderate decline in function. The doctor recognizes that fondaparinux is cleared by the kidney, and therefore monitoring the concentration of fondaparinux would be clinically informative, particularly while she is actively bleeding. The assay requested is the anti-factor Xa, using fondaparinux as the assay calibrator. The results show that the patient has a value well above the therapeutic range.

Explanation and Consequences

This case shows the importance of assessing renal function before administration of fondaparinux and the need to avoid the use of this anticoagulant in patients with moderate to severe renal impairment.

In addition, it shows that the appropriate monitoring assay is not the PTT but the anti-factor Xa assay calibrated with fondaparinux standards.

> ▶ Requesting an anti-factor Xa assay to monitor the effect of fondaparinux, but not indicating to the laboratory that the test is assessing the effect of fondaparinux. Unfractionated heparin and low molecular weight heparin can also be monitored by an anti-factor Xa assay. The laboratory uses fondaparinux to calibrate the assay when the anticoagulant effect of fondaparinux is being assessed; it uses low molecular weight heparin to calibrate the assay when the anticoagulant effect of low molecular weight heparin is being assessed; and it uses unfractionated heparin when the anticoagulant effect of unfractionated heparin is being measured. The laboratory must be made aware, therefore, that the requested test is to monitor the effect of fondaparinux.

Case with Error

An anti-factor Xa assay is requested for a patient receiving fondaparinux, but no information is provided to the clinical laboratory to indicate that fondaparinux is the anticoagulant that is being monitored. An assay is performed in the laboratory to measure the anti-factor Xa activity of low molecular weight heparin. An anti-factor Xa value is provided to the doctor that does not reflect the true anticoagulant status of the patient.

Explanation and Consequences

As noted in case 2, in Chapter 2 on monitoring unfractionated heparin therapy, the clinical laboratory must know if an anti-factor Xa assay is being requested to monitor unfractionated heparin, low molecular weight heparin, or fondaparinux. The potential consequence is that the doctor may inappropriately adjust the dosage of fondaparinux.

RESULT INTERPRETATION MISTAKES

▶ Failing to review and act upon a supratherapeutic or sub-therapeutic anti-factor Xa value in a patient being treated with fondaparinux in a timely fashion. The potential consequences for patients requiring anticoagulation with fondaparinux whose anti-factor Xa is not in the therapeutic range are bleeding (for anti-factor Xa values above the therapeutic range) and thrombosis (for anti-factor Xa values below the therapeutic range).

Case with Error

A patient being treated with therapeutic doses of fondaparinux develops significant bleeding from multiple sites. An anti-factor Xa assay for fondaparinux is performed, and the result is well above the therapeutic range. Unlike unfractionated heparin, which can be neutralized virtually completely by protamine, and low molecular weight heparin, which can be neutralized to a significant extent by protamine, protamine does not inactivate fondaparinux. Anecdotal reports of attempted reversal of fondaparinux-associated bleeding with recombinant factor VIIa exist, but no well accepted antidote to reduce fondaparinux-associated bleeding has been identified. Therefore, prompt action to treat a bleeding patient with an anti-factor Xa value above the therapeutic range is problematic for fondaparinux. However, an awareness that a supratherapeutic value for fondaparinux is a likely explanation for bleeding can limit the need to identify other potential causes for the bleeding.

Explanation and Consequences

This case highlights the lack of reversibility of fondaparinux and the watchful waiting that may be necessary in a bleeding patient treated with fondaparinux who has a supratherapeutic level of anti-factor Xa activity.

▶ Confusing the therapeutic range in the anti-factor Xa assay for fondaparinux (0.5–1.5 mcg/mL for a 7.5 mg daily dose) with that of the range for low molecular weight heparin (0.5–1.0 U/mL) and unfractionated heparin (0.3–0.7 U/mL).

Case with Error Averted

A patient treated with a 7.5 mg daily therapeutic dose of fondaparinux begins to develop significant hematomas with blood sample collection. An anti-factor Xa assay shows a value of 1.2 mcg/mL. This value is at first thought to be above the therapeutic range. The doctor inquires about the therapeutic range for fondaparinux from the clinical laboratory and learns that 1.2 is the number that could easily be perceived as supratherapeutic because 1.2 U/mL for unfractionated heparin or low molecular weight heparin would be supratherapeutic. The doctor is educated and understands that the observed anti-factor Xa level of 1.2 mcg/mL for her patient being treated with fondaparinux is within the therapeutic range. Another cause is pursued to explain the new hematomas.

Explanation and Consequences

In this case, the inquiry of the doctor about the therapeutic range prevented the incorrect conclusion that the anti-factor Xa level in this fondaparinux-treated patient was supratherapeutic and a possible explanation for the hematomas.

> ▶ Expecting a therapeutic anti-factor Xa level after treatment with a prophylactic fondaparinux dose. Treatment with a prophylactic dose of fondaparinux produces an anti-factor Xa level that is well below the therapeutic range.

Case with Error

A 52-year-old man receives a prophylactic dose of fondaparinux after orthopedic surgery on his knee. The doctor expects that this dosing will produce a value in the therapeutic range for the anti-factor Xa assay and requests the test in the absence of a true clinical need to do so. The result is subtherapeutic. However, no adjustment in fondaparinux dosing is made.

Explanation and Consequences

The mistake in this case was ordering a test to monitor the fondaparinux when the patient is receiving a prophylactic dose and is not bleeding. As with unfractionated heparin and low molecular weight heparin, prophylactic doses of fondaparinux do not produce values within the therapeutic range. The therapeutic range for fondaparinux has been established for patients receiving 7.5 mg daily of fondaparinux, which is the middle of the three therapeutic dose options for this anticoagulant (5, 7.5, and 10 mg).

OTHER MISTAKES

Not collecting a sample for anti-factor Xa monitoring of the patient treated with fondaparinux at the correct time after subcutaneous administration of the drug. The therapeutic effect of fondaparinux should be assessed after at least 3 hours post injection. Values before 3 hours may be different from those obtained after 3 hours. The half-life for fondaparinux is relatively long, so the timing of the blood sampling need not be as precise as for monitoring low molecular weight heparin. A misleading laboratory result could lead to inappropriate adjustment of the fondaparinux dose. It should be noted, however, that dosing of fondaparinux is not as precise as dosing of low molecular weight heparin. Patients less than 50 kg are recommended to receive 5 mg of fondaparinux daily; patients weighing between 50 and 100 kg are recommended to receive 7.5 mg of fondaparinux daily; and patients weighing more than 100 kg should receive 10 mg daily. Dosing with low molecular weight heparin is on a per kilogram basis, as is dosing with unfractionated heparin. Therefore, dose adjustments are far more commonly required with unfractionated heparin and low molecular weight heparin than for fondaparinux.

Case with Error

A bleeding patient treated with fondaparinux by subcutaneous injection is monitored with an assay for anti-factor Xa. A blood sample for this assay is collected 1 hour after the subcutaneous injection. The result of this test provides a value that does not represent the activity of fondaparinux that will appear in the circulation after 3 hours, and it should not be used for dose adjustment. The doctor is made aware of this fact when the laboratory learns the time interval between injection of the anticoagulant and sample collection for anticoagulant monitoring.

Explanation and Consequences

Unlike patients being treated with low molecular weight heparin, from whom samples should be collected 4 hours after subcutaneous injection, fondaparinux monitoring should be performed using samples collected not earlier than 3 hours and up to approximately 6 hours after subcutaneous injection. This will provide a value that is most appropriate for decision making about dose adjustment. The patient could have received a higher fondaparinux dose than needed had the physician acted upon the anti-factor Xa value obtained 1 hour after subcutaneous injection.

CONTROVERSY

It is not absolutely clear whether treatment with fondaparinux carries any risk for development of clinically significant HIT. There have been case reports of an occasional patient who may have developed heparin-induced thrombocytopenia following exposure to fondaparinux. Importantly, if these patients had any previous exposure to heparin or low molecular weight heparin in any form at any time, which was not known to the authors of these reports, fondaparinux may not have been the cause of the observed HIT.

STANDARDS OF CARE

■ Patients receiving fondaparinux who must be monitored for bleeding and thrombotic complications are evaluated using an anti-factor Xa assay with a therapeutic range for fondaparinux of 0.5–1.5 mcg/mL for patients receiving 7.5 mg of fondaparinux daily.

■ Subtherapeutic and supratherapeutic anti-factor Xa values must be recognized in a timely fashion, though it may be difficult to minimize the risk of bleeding if the value is supratherapeutic because there is no reversal agent for fondaparinux.

■ Samples collected for monitoring the effect of fondaparinux with an anti-factor Xa assay must not be collected before 3 hours from the time of the subcutaneous injection of the drug.

5 Monitoring of Anticoagulant Therapy in Patients Being Treated with Lepirudin or Argatroban

OVERVIEW

Direct thrombin inhibitors, which include lepirudin and argatroban, are commonly used anticoagulants in patients with HIT and in individuals tested for whatever reason and found to have antibodies to the heparin–platelet factor 4 complex in the absence of thrombocytopenia or thrombosis. These direct thrombin inhibitors are monitored with the standard PTT assay. Monitoring is especially important because neither of these compounds has an effective antidote to reverse over-anticoagulation. Monitoring is also made more difficult because these compounds also have an effect on the PT and, as a result, on the INR derived from it. In a typical patient with HIT transitioning from lepirudin or argatroban to warfarin, in an overlap phase during which time warfarin is present along with lepirudin or argatroban, there are special considerations necessary to obtain an INR that accurately reflects warfarin-induced anticoagulation. In addition, frequent monitoring of the PTT is highly recommended, especially if lepirudin is used in the presence of renal dysfunction and if argatroban is used in the presence of liver dysfunction.

TEST ORDERING MISTAKES

▶ Not monitoring the PTT frequently enough after the initiation of therapy with lepirudin or argatroban. Because lepirudin is cleared by the kidney, renal impairment can have a significant effect on the retention of lepirudin in the circulation. Reduced clearance of lepirudin can dramatically prolong the half-life for this anticoagulant, which has no known antidote. The safer choice is to avoid lepirudin in patients with any level of renal dysfunction. However, if lepirudin has been administered in a patient with decreased renal function, monitoring the prolongation of the PTT induced by lepirudin more than once per day may be informative to assess the risk for bleeding and the rate of return to therapeutic anticoagulation.

Argatroban is cleared by the liver, and, therefore, liver disease can reduce the rate at which argatroban is removed from the circulation. Unlike the situation with renal disease and lepirudin, however, it is common to use argatroban in patients with liver disease, but at a reduced dose. In patients with liver disease, monitoring of the PTT more than once per day to determine if the standard argatroban dose has been correctly reduced is essential to avoid under- or over-anticoagulation of the patient.

Case with Error

A 75-year-old man undergoes surgery to remove a bowel obstruction, and postoperatively he develops HIT, associated with a deep vein thrombosis. He has significant renal impairment, and tests for liver function show mild abnormalities. He is treated with argatroban at a dose of 2 mcg/kg/min. This results in a PTT of 95 seconds and bleeding from puncture sites. The dose of argatroban is reduced to 0.5 mcg/kg/min; the PTT shortens to 48 seconds; and the bleeding stops.

Explanation and Consequences

This case illustrates that argatroban can still be used in patients with liver disease with appropriate dose adjustments. Fortunately, the dose of argatroban was promptly adjusted to reduce the likelihood of major bleeding.

> ▶ Argatroban produces significant interference with the INR. Therefore, in patients being treated with argatroban and warfarin at the same time, with the intention to discontinue argatroban when a therapeutic effect of warfarin is achieved, the INR cannot be used to determine the warfarin effect. In such cases, the argatroban can be discontinued for 2 to 3 hours (the half-life is approximately 20 minutes), and the INR tested at that time. Because the patient might not be therapeutically anti-coagulated with warfarin, the removal of argatroban can result in thrombosis during this interval. Another option is to use a chromogenic assay for factor X to determine if warfarin has decreased the level of factor X to an expected concentration. Warfarin typically decreases factor X, along with factors II, VII, and IX. The chromogenic assay for factor X is not affected by argatroban. This permits testing for a warfarin effect while the patient is still receiving argatroban, and thereby anticoagulated with argatroban even if the warfarin effect is subtherapeutic at that time. A chromogenic factor X level of less than 45% has been recommended as adequate to permit discontinuation of argatroban and treatment with warfarin alone.

Lepirudin also influences the INR, but to a lesser extent than argatroban. If lepirudin is provided in a dose that prolongs the PTT into the lower end of the therapeutic range, it has a minimal effect on the INR. Therefore, in patients being treated with both lepirudin and warfarin, it is still possible to assess the extent of warfarin-induced anticoagulation with the INR and obviate the need for a chromogenic factor X assay.

Case with Error Averted

A 75-year-old stroke patient is being treated with lepirudin because of the development of HIT. The dose of lepirudin results in a PTT value approximately 2.5 times the mean of the normal range for the PTT. This is in the upper end of the therapeutic range for lepirudin. Warfarin is added with the intention to discontinue lepirudin when the warfarin produces a fully therapeutic anticoagulant effect. An INR obtained 5 days after the initiation of warfarin therapy is 12. The doctor learns that if the lepirudin dose is adjusted to produce a PTT in the lower end of the therapeutic range, a true INR that is not influenced by lepirudin can be obtained. With the adjustment in the dose of lepirudin to produce a therapeutic PTT value of 1.5 times the mean of the normal PTT range, the INR decreases to 2.8. With this information, the lepirudin is discontinued and the patient is maintained on warfarin alone. The INR in the presence of warfarin alone on the next day is 2.6.

Explanation and Consequences

Argatroban interferes with the INR in patients being treated with both argatroban and warfarin, no matter what dose of argatroban is used. This case shows that the dose of lepirudin can be adjusted within the therapeutic range for lepirudin, and not interfere with the INR, for patients receiving lepirudin and warfarin concomitantly. An appropriate decision was made regarding lepirudin discontinuation in this case because the value for the INR was interpretable and largely independent of interference from lepirudin.

The sixth case in Chapter 1 on monitoring warfarin anticoagulation also shows a case that illustrates the concept above.

RESULT INTERPRETATION MISTAKES

> ▶ Underdosing direct thrombin inhibitors in patients with both HIT and the lupus anticoagulant. In the rare patient with both HIT and a lupus anticoagulant, the PTT is prolonged before anticoagulation from the lupus anticoagulant. If the standard target range for the direct thrombin inhibitor of 1.5 to 2.5 times the mean of the normal PTT range is used to dose the direct thrombin inhibitor, an inadequate dose of the anticoagulant is likely to be provided. If the PT is not prolonged from the lupus anticoagulant, an increase in the PT to an arbitrarily accepted therapeutic range is one option to monitor direct thrombin inhibitors in these circumstances.

Case with Error

An 85-year-old man recently given unfractionated heparin for stroke develops HIT. The patient is also known to have a lupus anticoagulant and a prolonged PTT value on that basis. The patient is switched from unfractionated heparin to argatroban for anticoagulation. A major challenge exists for argatroban monitoring, however, because the lupus anticoagulant has prolonged the PTT almost into a range considered therapeutic for argatroban. When the standard therapeutic PTT range for argatroban of 1.5 to 2.5 times the mean of the normal PTT range is used to determine the argatroban dose, the argatroban dose is extremely low. For that reason, the PTT therapeutic range is then abandoned because it leads to inadequate anticoagulation with argatroban.

Explanation and Consequences

The doctor must decide upon an alternate plan for monitoring argatroban because the PTT therapeutic range is not useful. An arbitrary elevation in the PT, if it has been normal before argatroban therapy, can be used to establish a dosing plan for argatroban. However, it should be noted that monitoring argatroban with the PT is rarely performed, and for this reason, the therapeutic PT range that is chosen is arbitrary.

STANDARDS OF CARE

▨ Patients receiving lepirudin should be monitored frequently, typically more than once per day, especially during dose adjustment and if there is any indication of renal impairment.

▨ Patients receiving argatroban should also be monitored more than once per day, especially as the anticoagulant dose is adjusted and when argatroban is used in patients with liver disease.

▨ Patients being treated with argatroban and warfarin should ideally be monitored to assess warfarin-induced anticoagulation with a chromogenic factor X assay. Another option is to discontinue the argatroban for 2 to 3 hours and then perform the INR to assess the warfarin effect.

▨ Patients being treated with lepirudin and warfarin should be receiving lepirudin to prolong the PTT into the lower end of the therapeutic range to permit warfarin monitoring with the INR.

▨ Patients with both HIT and a lupus anticoagulant that prolongs the PTT, being treated with a direct thrombin inhibitor, cannot being monitored with the standard target PTT range for the direct thrombin inhibitors anticoagulation.

6 | Evaluation for Heparin-induced Thrombocytopenia

OVERVIEW

Heparin-induced thrombocytopenia or HIT is a highly prothrombotic condition, which can lead to arterial or venous thrombosis. A diagnosis of HIT indicates that antibodies are present to the heparin–platelet factor 4 complex; and thrombocytopenia exists to less than 50% of the patient's baseline platelet count, or there is a documented thrombosis. The thrombocytopenia in this condition is relatively modest, with values in the range of 40 000 to 80 000 per microliter. Importantly, the platelet count may not be decreased below the reference range. A patient who suffers a decline in platelet count from 600 000 per microliter to 300 000 per microliter has an equivalent risk for thrombosis as someone whose platelet count decreases from 150 000 per microliter to 75 000 per microliter. If the patient's platelet count decreases less than 4 days after exposure to heparin, it is unlikely that the patient has heparin-induced thrombocytopenia. The criteria known as the 4 T's to aid in the diagnosis of HIT refer to an appropriate level of Thrombocytopenia, appropriate Timing of the decline in the platelet count, the presence of Thrombosis, and the presence of other causes for Thrombocytopenia.

HIT-associated thromboses include deep vein thrombosis, pulmonary embolism, stroke, peripheral artery thrombosis and massive thrombosis with death. These poor clinical outcomes have in recent years resulted in a high vigilance state among physicians for this condition. There has been increased legal action against physicians who fail to recognize, demonstrate, and appropriately treat patients with HIT. The major challenge in this condition is that many patients will develop the antibody associated with HIT, which recognizes the heparin–platelet factor 4 complex, but they will not go on to develop thrombocytopenia or subsequently, thrombosis. The most commonly performed laboratory test for HIT is an enzyme-linked immunoassay, and recent improvements to this assay may better identify those patients who are at higher risk for thrombosis. Enzyme-linked immunoassays that detect immunoglobulin G (IgG) antibodies specifically to the heparin–platelet factor 4 complex have a high negative predictive value. IgG antibodies activate platelets in HIT, whereas IgM antibodies do not. In addition, IgM antibodies to the heparin–platelet 4 complex do not precede the appearance of IgG antibodies to the same target antigen. The best evidence for a diagnosis of HIT is a functional assay with washed platelets, and it is often used to confirm a diagnosis of HIT and better identify those patients with the antibody to the heparin–platelet factor 4 complex who will go on to develop thrombosis. This complex assay involving the use of radioactive serotonin is performed in very few clinical laboratories. The lack of availability of this assay in all but a few laboratories has made it impossible to use this test to make timely decisions regarding HIT diagnosis and therapy.

Because thrombocytopenia precedes thrombosis in HIT patients in the vast majority of cases, the platelet count is the major indicator that a patient with the antibody to the heparin–platelet factor 4 complex has an elevated thrombotic risk. The concern for both the high morbidity and mortality and the legal risk for missing a diagnosis of HIT has led to overtesting for antibodies to the heparin–platelet factor 4 complex. Overtesting commonly occurs in cases in which there is only a modest decline in the platelet count. Some physicians order the test for the antibody to the heparin–platelet factor 4 complex without performing a platelet count simply because of anticipated exposure to unfractionated heparin, and the fear that a previously acquired HIT associated antibody will initiate massive thrombosis. In some circumstances, such as the postoperative state following cardiac or vascular surgery, the platelet count decreases as part of the response to surgery and cannot be used effectively as an indicator of thrombotic risk. In situations when the platelet count cannot be used as an indicator of thrombotic risk, and an antibody to the heparin–platelet factor 4 complex is present, the concern for thrombosis commonly leads to the use of anticoagulants other than unfractionated heparin or low molecular weight heparin.

TEST ORDERING MISTAKES

> ▶ Failing to monitor the platelet count at least every third day in a hospitalized patient starting 4 days after the initial exposure to unfractionated heparin. The platelet count should be checked in patients who have had any exposure to unfractionated heparin, even if it is not provided as intravenous therapy. The platelet count can also decline, and antibodies to the heparin–platelet factor 4 complex can arise, in patients treated with low molecular weight heparin who have not been previously exposed to unfractionated heparin. However, the likelihood for the development of such antibodies is much less than that for patients exposed to unfractionated heparin.

A case with the error of inadequate platelet monitoring is described as the first case in Chapter 2 on the monitoring of unfractionated heparin.

> ▶ Ordering the test for antibodies to the heparin–platelet factor 4 complex when there is no meaningful decrease in platelet count (meaningful is less than 50% of baseline) and no thrombosis. A positive test result in this assay typically forces a change to an anticoagulant other than unfractionated heparin and low molecular weight heparin, and these are more expensive and less reversible anticoagulants.

Case with Error

A 71-year-old man is admitted for coronary artery bypass surgery. Because of anticipated exposure to unfractionated heparin during the surgery, the patient is tested upon admission for antibodies to the heparin–platelet factor 4 complex, and they are found to be present. The platelet count is 325 000 per microliter, which is well within the reference range, and the patient has a negative history for thrombosis. Major decisions must be made with regard to anticoagulation during and after bypass surgery because of the presence of the antibodies. This patient had been exposed to heparin previously, in an earlier hospitalization several months ago, and may have developed the antibodies at this time.

Explanation and Consequences

This case illustrates the problems associated with testing for antibodies to the heparin–platelet factor 4 complex when there is no indication to do so. If unfractionated heparin is used in surgery as planned, and thrombosis does arise, the surgeon and anesthesiologist will need to explain why they exposed the patient to heparin with the knowledge that the patient had antibodies to the heparin–platelet factor 4 complex. The consequences of this positive test are significant, resulting in major changes in anticoagulant use, which are of uncertain value because the patient has a normal platelet count and no evidence of thrombosis.

> ▶ Failing to order a test for antibodies to the heparin–platelet factor 4 complex in a nonthrombotic patient who has been exposed to unfractionated heparin or low molecular weight heparin who demonstrates (1) a decrease in platelet count to a level expected with HIT (approximately 50 000 per microliter as a mean value), (2) in a timeframe consistent with antibody production following exposure to heparin or low molecular weight heparin (4–15 days is common in the absence of an anamnestic response), and (3) no other apparent cause for thrombocytopenia.

Case with Error

A 48-year-old woman develops a significant pulmonary embolism and is being treated with unfractionated heparin. Her platelet count has declined to one-third of her baseline value, with the decline beginning 6 days after the initiation of heparin therapy. A nadir value is reached 12 days after the start of heparin therapy. A diagnosis of HIT is never considered. The patient continues treatment with unfractionated heparin, and then develops a lethal massive pulmonary embolism.

Explanation and Consequences

In this case, the thrombotic event resulted in mortality. Thrombosis associated with HIT is not infrequently catastrophic. This patient showed an appropriate decline of her platelet count at an appropriate rate which should have raised suspicion for HIT and provoke testing for this condition.

RESULT INTERPRETATION MISTAKES

> ▶ Failing to completely discontinue exposure to heparin and low molecular weight heparin in a patient who has antibodies to the heparin–platelet factor 4 complex, and failing to change the anticoagulation regimen to minimize the risk for thrombosis in such patients. Typically, this involves a change to an anticoagulant other than unfractionated heparin or low molecular weight heparin and avoidance of monotherapy with warfarin until the platelet count rises into the reference range.

Case with Error

A 67-year-old man develops HIT. The doctor recognizes the condition and discontinues the unfractionated heparin and initiates warfarin therapy. Within 1 day of the initiation of warfarin therapy, in the absence of any other anticoagulant, when the platelet count remains low at 63 000 per microliter, the patient develops bilateral deep vein thrombosis.

Explanation and Consequences

This case illustrates the danger of initiating monotherapy with warfarin for patients with HIT. Warfarin decreases the synthesis of four coagulation factors, as well as two natural anticoagulants, protein C and protein S. In addition, the full effect of warfarin anticoagulation appears only several days after it is initiated. Therefore, warfarin monotherapy is ineffective in the early course of warfarin treatment. Warfarin can be used as long-term monotherapy for patients with heparin–antiplatelet factor 4 antibodies if it is initiated in the presence of an anticoagulant suitable for patients with HIT, such as argatroban and lepirudin.

> ▶ Treating a patient with platelets who has a positive test for antibodies to the heparin–platelet factor 4 complex. In such patients, the antibodies can induce the generation of platelet aggregates large enough to occlude major arteries, and the transfusion of platelets increases the risk for such catastrophic thromboses.

Case with Error

A 67-year-old woman develops a right-sided deep vein thrombosis that extends into the inferior vena cava. She is hospitalized and is treated with unfractionated heparin. Over the course of the next 10 days, she develops thrombocytopenia with a platelet count of 32 000 per microliter and a positive test for heparin–platelet factor 4 antibodies. The doctor is concerned about the risk of spontaneous bleeding with such a low platelet count and transfuses the patient with 6 units of random donor platelet concentrates. Despite the change in anticoagulation from unfractionated heparin to argatroban, the patient develops an arterial thrombosis in her right forearm.

Explanation and Consequences

The use of platelets is highly contraindicated in patients with heparin–platelet factor 4 antibodies. These antibodies can activate platelets, and thereby induce platelet clumping that occludes blood vessels large enough to generate clinically significant thrombosis. This patient ultimately lost a portion of one digit as a result of the thrombosis.

OTHER MISTAKES

▶ The failure of the laboratory to provide the results for the test for antibodies to the heparin–platelet factor 4 complex in a timely fashion. Delay in the processing of samples for this test forces the treating physician observing a decrease in platelet count consistent with HIT to decide whether to switch to more expensive anticoagulant therapy without a knowledge of the test results. The practical challenge for small laboratories is that the test for antibodies to the heparin–platelet factor 4 complex is often not performed on-site, but is sent to an outside laboratory. It is not uncommon in these situations to wait several days for a test result, despite the fact that there is an urgent need in such cases to make a major decision about appropriate anticoagulant use.

Case with Error

A patient being treated with unfractionated heparin in a 200-bed community hospital shows a decline in platelet count consistent with the presence of HIT. A test for the presence of antibodies to the heparin–platelet factor 4 complex is not available in the clinical laboratory of this hospital. The sample is sent to an outside laboratory for this test, and the results will be available in 3 days. The doctor treating the patient makes a decision to continue treatment with unfractionated heparin until the result of the test for the antibodies is available. While waiting for this test result, the patient develops a life-threatening pulmonary embolism.

Explanation and Consequences

This is a common occurrence because the assay for antibodies to the heparin–platelet factor 4 complex is not performed in the clinical laboratories of most hospitals. This forces doctors to decide whether to switch a patient from heparin to a much more expensive anticoagulant. Making such a switch is the safer course of action, but it is an inconvenience to the patient, if it is necessary at all, and an added expense to the hospital.

CONTROVERSY

Monitoring the platelet count of patients who are not in the hospital and are receiving low molecular weight heparin at home. These patients are at some measurable risk for HIT, although it varies to some extent with their underlying clinical circumstances. For example, patients recovering from orthopedic surgery are at higher risk for development of antibodies to the heparin–platelet factor 4 complex than are patients with non-surgical conditions. The logistical challenge of obtaining platelet counts for patients at home receiving low molecular weight heparin has resulted in acceptance of low molecular weight heparin treatment in the absence of platelet counts.

STANDARDS OF CARE

■ A platelet count should be performed at least every third day in a hospitalized patient receiving unfractionated heparin beginning 4 days after initial heparin exposure.

■ A test for antibodies to the heparin–platelet factor 4 complex should be performed for a patient who has been exposed to unfractionated heparin or low molecular weight heparin and who demonstrates a decrease in platelet count that could be indicative of HIT.

■ A test for antibodies to the heparin–platelet factor 4 complex should not be ordered when there is no meaningful decrease in platelet count (ie, less than 50% of baseline) and no thrombosis.

■ Exposure to heparin and low molecular weight heparin must be immediately discontinued in a patient who has antibodies to the heparin–platelet factor 4 complex.

■ The anticoagulation regimen in a patient with antibodies to the heparin–platelet factor 4 complex must be appropriate to minimize the risk for thrombosis.

■ Platelet transfusions must be avoided in a patient who has a positive test for antibodies to the heparin–platelet factor 4 complex.

Evaluation of Prolongations of the PT and the PTT and Assessment for Deficiencies of Coagulation Factors

OVERVIEW

There are many errors associated with the orders for coagulation factors. PT and PTT prolongations may be a result of congenital deficiencies of one or more coagulation factors or from a host of acquired conditions associated with inhibitors or low levels of the coagulation factors. It is essential to diagnose the cause of a prolonged PT and PTT to determine the correct treatment, if one is needed. This often requires the determination of selected coagulation factor levels. It is a common mistake to replace factors by infusing the patient with fresh-frozen plasma and not identify the cause of the factor deficiencies and the associated prolongations of the PT and/or PTT.

It is the rare physician who recalls which factors are associated with only a prolonged PTT, only a prolonged PT, or a prolongation of both the PT and the PTT. Generally speaking, the factors associated with a prolonged PTT and a normal PT are the hours in the workday morning, 8 o'clock, 9 o'clock, but not 10 o'clock because it is a coffee break, 11 o'clock, and 12 noon. Thus, deficiencies of factors VIII, IX, XI, and XII are associated with a prolonged PTT in the presence of a normal PT. The factor associated with a prolonged PT in the presence of a normal PTT is factor VII, or the month of July when new residents appear on the staff. The factors in the common pathway of the coagulation cascade, when deficient, most often prolong the PT and the PTT, though the PT is affected more than the PTT. These common pathway factors can be remembered as the smallest denominations of paper currency in the United States; namely, the $1 bill, the $2 bill, the $5 bill, and the $10 bill. Thus, deficiencies of factors I (fibrinogen), II, V, and X commonly prolong both the PT and the PTT.

TEST ORDERING MISTAKES

▶ Ordering the incorrect coagulation factors from lack of knowledge about which coagulation factor deficiencies are associated with a PT prolongation and which coagulation factor deficiencies are associated with a PTT prolongation. For a PTT prolongation with a normal PT value, the most commonly identified factor deficiencies to consider are factors VIII, IX, XI, and XII. For a PT prolongation with a normal PTT value, the most important consideration is a deficiency of factor VII. Deficiencies of fibrinogen (factor I) and factors II, V, and X usually prolong both the PT and PTT. However, mild deficiencies in these factors may prolong only the PT.

Case with Error

The patient has a prolonged PTT and a consistently normal PT. The doctor orders all of the coagulation factors to evaluate the prolonged PTT.

Explanation and Consequences

A normal PT makes deficiencies of factors II, V, X, and VII unlikely, and therefore, these coagulation factor assays will not necessarily be informative. In this case, the clinical laboratory spent its resources, hundreds of dollars, and hours of time, unnecessarily. This delayed the results for tests that were of true clinical importance.

> ▶ Ordering coagulation factor assays while a patient is receiving warfarin. Patients receiving warfarin will have deficiencies of factors II, VII, IX, and X, and there is rarely any need to order factor assays to demonstrate these deficiencies in warfarin-treated patients.

Case with Error

The doctor sees that the INR is 6.3 in a patient receiving warfarin who has a long history of remaining within the therapeutic INR range of 2 to 3. She orders factor assays to explain the INR that is above the therapeutic range.

Explanation and Consequences

For the occasional elevation above the therapeutic range, testing for factors II, VII, IX, and X in a patient treated with warfarin is unnecessary. The clinical laboratory spent time and money to perform testing that did not provide clinical value.

> ▶️Ordering coagulation factor assays while a patient is receiving a direct thrombin inhibitor, most commonly argatroban or lepirudin. Thrombin, factor IIa, is near the very bottom of the coagulation cascade. Therefore, for all clot-based assays of coagulation factors, direct thrombin inhibitors will significantly interfere with these tests and provide uninterpretable results for the coagulation factors.

Case with Error

The doctor finds a prolonged PTT and prolonged PT in a patient being treated with argatroban. To further evaluate these prolongations, the doctor orders factors II, V, VII, X, VIII, IX, XI, and XII. All of the coagulation factor values are low.

Explanation and Consequences

Anticoagulants that inhibit the coagulation cascade at the bottom of the coagulation pathway, especially inhibitors of thrombin, will result in falsely low levels for all coagulation factors above this point in the cascade. Not only did the clinical laboratory spend time and money performing unnecessary tests but also there is a danger that the doctor unnecessarily provides transfusions or factor concentrates that can present infectious risk or thrombotic risk and be very costly.

> ▶️Confusing factor V with the factor V Leiden mutation. For patients who are bleeding and being evaluated for a factor V deficiency, the correct test is the factor V assay. For patients who have experienced thrombosis, the correct test is the factor V Leiden.

Case with Error

The patient has a thrombotic event, and the doctor orders an assay for factor V.

Explanation and Consequences

The level of factor V provides information on the amount of factor V present and an assessment of the risk for bleeding rather than the risk for thrombosis. This patient is being denied an assessment for the most common thrombotic risk factor among Caucasians because an incorrect test was ordered.

> ▶Confusing factor II (prothrombin) with the prothrombin 20210 mutation. For patients who are bleeding and being evaluated for a factor II deficiency, the correct test is the factor II or prothrombin assay. For patients who have experienced thrombosis, the correct test is the assay for the prothrombin 20210 mutation.

Case with Error

The patient has a thrombotic event, and the doctor orders an assay for factor II.

Explanation and Consequences

The level of factor II provides information on the amount of factor II present and an assessment of the risk for bleeding rather than the risk for thrombosis. Similar to the case above, this patient is denied an assessment for the second most common thrombotic risk factor among Caucasians because an incorrect test was ordered.

> ▶ Confusing factor IX with factor XI. The reversal of the *X* and the *I* can result in major errors in treatment that are expensive and can have serious adverse effects. For example, many factor XI–deficient patients need no treatment at all, and factor IX–deficient patients are often given expensive recombinant factor IX concentrate.

Case with Error

The PTT is prolonged and an assay for factor XI is ordered instead of an assay for factor IX, which is the desired assay for this patient. A low value of 6% is obtained for factor XI, but the patient has no bleeding. It is common for many factor XI–deficient patients to not bleed even when challenged. This patient is treated before surgery with fresh-frozen plasma to reduce the risk of expected bleeding because of the low value for factor XI. No assay for factor IX is ever performed.

Explanation and Consequences

A careful review of orders to make sure that factor IX and factor XI are not confused is very important because it can lead to inappropriate transfusions. Unnecessary transfusions present infectious risks and other potential complications, depending upon the product that is transfused.

> ▶ Confusing factor II with factor XI. It is important to remember that the correct numbering system for coagulation factors involves the use of Roman numerals. If a regular Arabic number (that is 11) is used to identify the number of the coagulation factor, an assay for factor II is often performed in the clinical laboratory.

Case with Error

The doctor orders a single coagulation factor assay for factor 11, in the absence of other factors. The technologist in the laboratory is not sure if this represents factor II or factor XI.

Explanation and Consequences

The incorrect use of Arabic numbers (11) instead of Roman numerals (XI) creates confusion and can lead to the performance of a factor II assay instead of the desired test for factor XI. A potential consequence in this case is that the patient has a true deficiency of factor XI that is overlooked because an assay for factor II was performed instead.

RESULT INTERPRETATION MISTAKES

Treating all coagulation factor deficiencies with fresh-frozen plasma as a source of the deficient factor. It should first be understood that not all factor deficiencies are associated with bleeding. Patients with even complete deficiencies of factor XII do not experience bleeding. Many patients with a significant factor VII or factor XI deficiency also do not bleed. The treatment for factor deficiencies depends upon the cause and the risk for bleeding. Many physicians incorrectly do not bother to determine if a factor deficiency is a result of an inherited factor deficiency, a result of anticoagulation, a component of a physiologic or pathologic process such as disseminated intravascular coagulation, or a consequence of liver disease. The treatment for a deficiency of the same coagulation factor can be very different in different clinical settings.

Case with Error

A neurosurgeon sees a patient who is undergoing coagulation testing with a PT and a PTT before a surgery to resect bilateral Schwannomas. The PT value is persistently prolonged in three assays over several weeks with a normal PTT in each case. Two hours before the surgery, the patient is given 2 units of fresh-frozen plasma, and there is no excess operative bleeding. On postoperative day 1, 2 more units of fresh-frozen plasma are infused. In the continued absence of bleeding, the fresh-frozen plasma infusions are then discontinued. On postoperative day 2, the patient experiences significant intracranial hemorrhage at the surgical sites bilaterally and suffers permanent major neurologic impairment.

Explanation and Consequences

This patient was found to have a congenitally low level of factor VII that was 30% to 40% of the normal level. Because this cause for the PT prolongation in this patient was never identified, and the patient was instead transfused with fresh-frozen plasma to overcome the PT prolongation with no investigation into its cause, the frequency and duration of fresh-frozen plasma transfusions were greatly underestimated, and they were discontinued prematurely. This resulted in the adverse outcome. A thorough evaluation of the cause of the prolonged PT before surgery would have permitted the development of a treatment plan more likely to be successful.

> ▶ Confusing a low level of a PTT-related coagulation factor (factors VIII, IX, XI, and XII) caused by a lupus anticoagulant with a congenital deficiency of 1 of these 4 factors. For example, confusing a patient with a lupus anticoagulant who has low levels of one or more PTT-related coagulation factors with a patient who has factor VIII deficiency can result in the infusion of expensive and potentially prothrombotic coagulation factor concentrates when they are completely unnecessary.

Case with Error

The doctor sees a patient who has a prolonged PTT. A PTT mixing was not ordered. Instead, factors VIII, IX, XI, and XII were all requested because of the known association of deficiencies of these factors with a prolonged PTT. All of the factors tested are low, and the conclusion by the doctor is that the patient has multiple congenital factor deficiencies.

Explanation and Consequences

The lupus anticoagulant usually inhibits more than one of the PTT-related coagulation factors, and this becomes apparent when all four of the PTT-related factors are measured using the same sample. The PTT mixing study is useful to identify an inhibitor, such as the lupus anticoagulant. The most common cause of a prolonged PTT that fails to normalize in a PTT mixing study is a lupus anticoagulant. The appropriate conclusion is that the patient has a lupus anticoagulant and not multiple congenital factor deficiencies, as the lupus anticoagulant is an inhibitor in PTT-based factor assays. The lupus anticoagulant is not associated with a bleeding risk, but it can be a risk factor for thrombosis. Treatments to replace factors that appear to be deficient, but are not truly deficient, in a patient with a lupus anticoagulant expose the patient to the risks of unnecessary transfusion.

▶ Concluding that slight elevations in the PT or the PTT are always clinically insignificant. This is a difficult circumstance because in most cases, minor elevations of a few seconds above the upper limit of normal for the PT and the PTT are indeed not often associated with a significant predisposition for bleeding. However, for the patient who has a single factor deficiency, such as a deficiency of factor IX, a persistent slight prolongation of the PTT may be associated with a congenitally low level of factor IX between 20% and 30%. If such a patient were taken to surgery and not provided with factor IX preoperatively, excess bleeding is likely to occur. Therefore, in the absence of a clear explanation for a slight elevation in the PT or the PTT, appropriate factor assays may be informative to identify single congenital factor deficiencies that can predispose the patient to bleeding.

Case with Error

The doctor orders a coagulation evaluation before surgery and finds a PTT that is prolonged only 3 seconds over the upper limit of normal. The doctor concludes that this slight elevation in the PTT presents no increased bleeding risk for surgery. The patient undergoes surgery and experiences a massive hemorrhage during the procedure. After surgery, a prolonged PTT evaluation reveals that the patient has a factor IX level of 33%, which is well below normal and requires treatment perioperatively to increase the level of factor IX and prevent bleeding.

Explanation and Consequences

It is not uncommon for certain coagulation testing instruments and test reagents to require a very decreased concentration of a coagulation factor to be present before the PTT becomes elevated above normal. Thus, it is possible for the factor IX level to be 33%, which would predispose to excess bleeding with surgery, and have a PTT value which is only slightly elevated, or even within the upper limit of the reference range. This case illustrates why slight but persistent elevations in the PT or PTT can be clinically significant and why they require an evaluation to determine the cause of the mild prolongations.

> ▶ Attempting to completely normalize the PT and the PTT in the patient who has liver disease and concomitantly a deficiency of multiple coagulation factors. In patients with liver disease, slight prolongations of the PT and the PTT are rarely associated with an increased predisposition to bleed. In such patients, attempts to bring the PT and the PTT within the reference range, rather than leaving them slightly above the upper limit of normal, often results in volume overload. If the patient has a prolonged PT and PTT on the basis of liver disease alone, minor elevations in the PT and PTT are often well tolerated. Therefore, it is not appropriate to continue to transfuse fresh-frozen plasma to fully normalize the PT and the PTT in the liver disease patient, who is not bleeding.

Case with Error

A patient has laboratory parameters consistent with cirrhosis and a clinical history of many years of excess ethanol intake. The doctor is interested in performing a liver biopsy. In anticipation of the biopsy, a PT is ordered and is found to be elevated. To minimize the risk for bleeding during the biopsy, the patient is transfused with fresh-frozen plasma. The PT fails to completely normalize and remains 2 to 3 seconds above the upper limit of normal, despite the administration of 20 units of fresh-frozen plasma over 2 days. The patient now experiences volume overload and has difficulty breathing.

Explanation and Consequences

In patients with liver disease who have PT prolongations as a result of decreased production of coagulation factors by the liver, massive amounts of transfusion can be given without fully normalizing the PT, as in this case. The amount of fresh-frozen plasma given to this patient was substantial and not surprisingly associated with volume overload and its complications.

> ▶ Failing to understand that the reference ranges for coagulation factors in children may be different from the reference ranges for coagulation factors in adults. For several factors, the reference ranges for children are lower than they are for adults. In addition, the age at which the adult reference range becomes relevant varies with the individual coagulation factor or natural anticoagulant. Because of this, children should be evaluated for deficiencies using the appropriate age-adjusted reference range.

Case with Error

A 6-month-old child develops a significant venous thrombosis in the absence of a catheter. A test panel for hypercoagulability is performed and reveals low values for protein C, protein S, and antithrombin. The protein C value is especially below the reference range included in the report. The doctor mistakenly concludes that the patient has multiple congenital deficiencies of natural anticoagulants and on that basis developed venous thrombosis.

Explanation and Consequences

The reference ranges for several coagulation factors and natural anticoagulants for children do not match those of adults. In most cases, the reference ranges for children are lower than those for adults. For that reason, to correctly interpret test results for protein C, protein S, and antithrombin in this case, the patient's results must be compared to an age-appropriate reference range. A child does not reach an adult-level reference range for protein C until sometime between the ages of 9 and 12 years. The potential consequence is that this child would be considered hypercoagulable on the basis of a deficiency of protein C. This could result in unnecessary prophylactic anticoagulation during periods of increased thrombotic risk and testing of family members for protein C deficiency.

ERRORS WITHIN THE CLINICAL LABORATORY

▶ The clinical laboratory not performing factor assays at multiple plasma dilutions to reveal a factor inhibitor, if it is present. A coagulation factor level may be low because there is decreased synthesis of the factor or because there is an inhibitor of the factor. This differentiation is essential because the treatment for a factor deficiency is usually very different from the treatment for a factor inhibitor. For example, a simple inherited deficiency of factor VIII is often treated with factor VIII concentrate, whereas a deficiency resulting from a clinically apparent factor VIII inhibitor may be treated with recombinant factor VIIa.

Case with Error

A patient with a prolonged PTT and no history of bleeding presents for a preoperative evaluation. PTT-related coagulation factors (VIII, IX, XI, and XII) are measured. The laboratory performs the PTT-related coagulation factor assays using a single dilution of the patient's plasma (1:10) to establish the values for each of the factors tested. The results for all of the PTT-related factors are low. In addition, a lupus anticoagulant is ordered and is found to be positive. The doctor concludes that there are deficiencies of all four of these factors and begins to consider options for preoperative transfusion to minimize bleeding perioperatively.

Explanation and Consequences

Assays for coagulation factors in a clinical laboratory should be performed at multiple plasma dilutions. It is common to measure a coagulation factor using plasma dilutions of 1:10, 1:20, and 1:40. When there is an inhibitor in the sample, such as a lupus anticoagulant in this case, the lowest dilution (1:10 here) shows an erroneously low value, because the inhibitor is most potent at low dilutions of plasma. The factor values at the higher plasma dilutions show a decreased impact of the inhibitor and more accurately reflect the true level of the coagulation factor in the plasma. It is common for laboratories to report the coagulation factor level detected at the highest dilution (1:40 in this case) as the true value. In this case, only one low dilution was assayed, and this resulted in the reporting of falsely low values for the four PTT-related coagulation factors. The danger of this misinterpretation is that the patient could be given a diagnosis of one or more factor deficiencies and be treated unnecessarily for a factor deficiency with factor concentrates or blood products that carry infectious and/or thrombotic risks.

> ▶ The failure to remove heparin, if present, from a plasma specimen before performance of coagulation factor assays and inhibitor testing. Heparin can be removed from a plasma sample by the addition of a heparin-degrading enzyme to the sample. This will remove the anticoagulant effect of heparin from the sample.

Case with Error

A patient being treated with heparin for a pulmonary embolism is evaluated for a lupus anticoagulant using a PTT-based assay sensitive to the lupus anticoagulant. The test result is positive. The laboratory fails to remove the heparin from the sample before performing the test for the lupus anticoagulant that is positive. The doctor concludes that the patient has a lupus anticoagulant.

Explanation and Consequences

Heparin can significantly interfere with many assays in the coagulation laboratory. In this example, a PTT-based assay for the lupus anticoagulant suffers interference from heparin, and therefore, no conclusion can be made about the presence of a lupus anticoagulant. If heparin is removed from the sample, for example, using a heparin-degrading enzyme, the assay for the lupus anticoagulant can be interpreted accurately, because a false-positive result from heparin in the sample is no longer a concern. A false-positive test for a lupus anticoagulant could mistakenly identify the patient as having an increased risk for thrombosis.

STANDARDS OF CARE

■ Prolongations of the PTT and the PT should lead to the appropriate selection of coagulation factor assays or inhibitors to explain the prolongations identified.

■ Factor inhibitors must be differentiated from factor deficiencies.

■ Reduced levels of coagulation factors produced by direct thrombin inhibitors, such as argatroban and lepirudin, should not be confused with true deficiencies of coagulation factors.

■ The correct numbering terminology for coagulation factor numbers involves the use of Roman numerals.

■ Factor V and prothrombin tests must be carefully differentiated from the assays for factor V Leiden and the prothrombin 20210 mutations, respectively.

■ Treatment of coagulation factor deficiencies should be directed by the cause of the deficiency and not by replacing the deficient coagulation factors with fresh-frozen plasma without determining the cause of the deficiency.

■ Determination of the cause of a slight prolongation of the PT or PTT must be made to include consideration of a clinically significant factor deficiency.

■ Age-adjusted reference ranges must be used in the assessment of children for deficiencies of coagulation factors and natural anticoagulants.

■ The coagulation laboratory must clearly differentiate a lupus anticoagulant from PTT-related factor deficiencies.

■ The coagulation laboratory must remove heparin from samples in which it is present when clot-based coagulation and inhibitor assays need to be performed with the samples.

8 Evaluation for Disseminated Intravascular Coagulation

OVERVIEW

Disseminated intravascular coagulation (DIC) results from a stimulus that activates coagulation and thereby consumes platelets and coagulation factors in small blood vessels. The depletion of platelets and coagulation factors in capillaries is the reason why DIC is associated with bleeding rather than thrombosis in the vast majority of cases. Despite the fact that DIC is commonly encountered, the diagnosis of this condition can be very challenging. The parameters that change in patients with DIC, including an elevation in the D-dimer, which is of great importance in establishing a diagnosis of DIC, are similarly altered in a variety of other conditions. There is no single test that specifically indicates the presence of DIC. As a further diagnostic complication, the D-dimer assay can be performed by multiple methodologies that have different reference ranges. Some D-dimer tests are more complex to perform than others. For this reason, a single clinical laboratory may offer one method during the day and another method at other times. This can lead to significant confusion among physicians using the laboratory regarding the diagnosis of DIC because it is not always clear which assay was used to quantify the D-dimer. The treatment of a bleeding episode in DIC is replacement therapy with blood products containing the consumed components. Blood products may successfully stop a bleeding episode in a DIC patient, but they may also be ineffective. The inappropriate use of large numbers of blood products to stop a bleeding episode in a patient with an untreatable underlying cause for DIC should be avoided.

TEST ORDERING MISTAKES

▶ Ordering too many tests to establish a diagnosis of DIC. In DIC, there are many changes that can be detected in the blood. For example, complexes of thrombin and antithrombin are formed in DIC. Although assays are available for the measurement of thrombin–antithrombin complexes, these are impractical for performance at all times, even if they are available in the laboratory. A commonly used panel of tests useful for the diagnosis of DIC in a patient with an identified stimulus for DIC includes a platelet count (commonly decreased in acute DIC), a D-dimer assay (typically elevated in DIC), and a PT (usually prolonged in acute DIC). In addition, a peripheral blood smear (for schistocytes) and a fibrinogen test (most commonly serial fibrinogens to show that the fibrinogen value is decreasing) may be informative. The fibrinogen level is increased above normal, as part of the acute-phase response, by many of the stimuli for DIC. This is why a single fibrinogen test that is often normal in DIC can be uninformative. The D-dimer assay provides logistical advantages over the assay for fibrinogen degradation products (FDP), but an elevated FDP result can also be used to provide evidence of clot formation and clot degradation in DIC.

Case with Error

A 36-year-old woman with pneumonia resulting from a gram-negative infection begins to bleed from puncture sites and develops spontaneous bruising. An evaluation for DIC is performed and the following tests are ordered: platelet count, PT, PTT, fibrinogen, peripheral blood smear, D-dimer, FDP, protein C, protein S, and antithrombin. The results of the tests strongly support a diagnosis of DIC.

Explanation and Consequences

The tests in this assessment for DIC include three natural anticoagulants, namely protein C, protein S, and antithrombin. Although these proteins decrease in patients with acute DIC, they are not simple tests, are relatively expensive, and usually do not add diagnostic information when considering DIC as a possibility. In addition, this test panel includes assays for both D-dimer and FDP. The test for D-dimer is preferred, and the assay for FDP, when a test for D-dimer is already included, is unnecessary. The consequences of this excessive testing are the unnecessary expenditure of technologist's time and the laboratory's budget for test reagents.

RESULT INTERPRETATION MISTAKES

Confusing DIC with liver disease. In both DIC and liver disease, it is not uncommon to find a decreased platelet count, an elevated D-dimer, and an elevated PT. These changes occur by different mechanisms in the two disorders. In the absence of abnormalities in liver function tests, there is minimal difficulty in differentiating DIC from liver disease. However, when liver function tests are clearly abnormal, it may be difficult or impossible to determine if the laboratory changes are attributable to liver disease, DIC, or both. Severe liver failure is a known stimulus for DIC, so the presence of both abnormalities at the same time is a strong possibility.

Case with Error

A 42-year-old man suffering from liver disease produced by years of ethanol abuse is evaluated with routine blood tests. He is found to have a low platelet count, an elevated PT, and an elevated D-dimer. His liver function tests are markedly abnormal. The abnormalities in this patient with liver disease can be explained by a large spleen that sequesters platelets, a decreased mass of hepatocytes to synthesize coagulation factors, and a decreased ability of the reticuloendothelial cells in the liver to clear D-dimers from the circulation. DIC may also be present because these laboratory test results are characteristic findings in patients with DIC. In DIC, however, the changes observed occur as a result of consumption of platelets and coagulation factors and the formation and degradation of clots in the microcirculation. The doctor continues to order additional tests in the hopes of differentiating liver disease from DIC in this patient.

Explanation and Consequences

It has been suggested that an elevated level of factor VIII is associated more with liver disease than with DIC. However, this assay and others that have been proposed to convincingly differentiate liver disease from DIC are helpful in a small percentage of cases. In cases like the one described above, bleeding episodes would be treated with platelet concentrates and fresh-frozen plasma whether the diagnosis is hepatic failure or DIC. The performance of additional laboratory testing to differentiate these two disorders is likely to be nonproductive.

▶ Overlooking a diagnosis of compensated DIC. This can be a challenging diagnosis because, with the exception of an elevated D-dimer or FDP, the other major parameters of the DIC panel can be normal. Increased platelet production in the bone marrow can compensate for a low-grade consumption of platelets in DIC. Similarly, increased synthesis of coagulation factors in the liver can compensate for a low-grade consumption of coagulation factors in DIC. The potential danger of overlooking compensated DIC is that a minor challenge to such a patient, like an infection, can greatly reduce the compensatory actions of the bone marrow and the liver. This will result in the rapid appearance of significantly abnormal values for both the platelet count and the PT. It is reasonable to make the diagnosis of compensated DIC in retrospect, when the compensatory effects are no longer present.

Case with Error

A 54-year-old man carries a diagnosis of prostate cancer, which was identified 3 years earlier. As per his wishes, he has not been treated for the disorder. His platelet count is 150 000 per microliter, which is at the lower end of the reference range. His PT value is 13.0 seconds, which is reported to be at the upper limit of the reference range and still normal. He is found to have a slight increase in his D-dimer level. The patient develops a severe viral upper respiratory illness. Within days of the clinical appearance of the infection, the patient's platelet count decreases to 80 000 per microliter, and his PT increases to 16.3 seconds. The D-dimer level increases slightly. No diagnosis is made by the doctor.

Explanation and Consequences

One explanation for the findings in this case are that the patient's prostate cancer has been a stimulus for a chronic DIC that has been compensated for with increased platelet production and increased coagulation factor synthesis. The respiratory illness in this patient impairs the compensatory responses, and this raises the strong possibility that the patient has been experiencing a compensated form of DIC.

> ▶ Unless there are other reasons to do so, treatment of the patient with acute DIC who is not bleeding, using blood products to normalize a low platelet count (with platelet concentrates) or an elevated PT (with fresh-frozen plasma) or a low fibrinogen (with cryoprecipitate).

Case with Error

A patient with a fetal death in utero has changes in laboratory tests consistent with a diagnosis of acute DIC. However, she is experiencing no bleeding. To normalize the laboratory values, the doctor transfuses the patient with platelets, fresh-frozen plasma, and cryoprecipitate.

Explanation and Consequences

In patients with DIC who have a treatable underlying cause and no bleeding, the preferred option is to avoid transfusion of blood components unless bleeding occurs and remove the stimulus for DIC. Because there was no bleeding in this patient, and delivery of a stillborn fetus was highly likely to remove the cause of her DIC, treatment with blood products was unnecessary and exposed her to the risks associated with receiving blood components.

▶ The expectation that it is possible to stop a bleeding episode associated with an underlying DIC stimulus that cannot be effectively treated. For example, patients with pancreatic cancer who develop DIC are highly unlikely to have the stimulus for DIC removed. On the other hand, a woman with DIC as a result of a fetal death in utero can rapidly recover from DIC upon delivery of the stillborn fetus. Thoughtful use of blood products is essential in the bleeding patient with DIC because it is possible to greatly deplete the hospital supply of platelet concentrates, fresh-frozen plasma, and cryoprecipitate for a patient with DIC and an untreatable underlying disorder.

Case with Error

An 85-year-old man with metastatic lung cancer develops severe DIC and begins to bleed profusely from multiple sites. He is treated with 6 units of random donor platelets, 2 units of fresh-frozen plasma, and 8 units of cryoprecipitate. This treatment fails to stop the bleeding. A second round of the same blood components is administered, but the bleeding persists. The doctor decides to continue transfusions until all bleeding is stopped.

Explanation and Consequences

This case illustrates a patient with intractable DIC and an untreatable underlying illness as a stimulus for the DIC. When such patients have a major bleeding episode, it may be impossible to stop severe bleeding with blood component therapy. Continued use of blood products for such a patient may deprive other patients who might benefit from them of blood components.

OTHER MISTAKES

Clinical laboratories can use a variety of test methodologies for measurement of D-dimer. This test is used in the diagnosis of DIC and to rule out, when negative, venous thrombosis. A negative enzyme-linked immunoassay for D-dimer has long been the gold standard to rule out pulmonary embolism or deep vein thrombosis in the outpatient presenting for evaluation. The most widely used precursor assay of the enzyme-linked D-dimer immunoassay is a latex bead agglutination test. This assay has less sensitivity for the D-dimer than the enzyme-linked immunoassay, but it is extremely easy to perform. Because the enzyme-linked immunoassay is more technically complex, many clinical laboratories offer this higher sensitivity enzyme-linked immunoassay D-dimer measurement during the day, and switch to a latex agglutination test for the evening and night shifts in the laboratory. To add to the confusion, D-dimer assays by different methodologies can have different thresholds to determine when the test is positive. It can be extremely confusing to physicians who use a laboratory with multiple D-dimer assays to know which assay was performed on the samples collected from their patients, and because of this problem, to correctly interpret the test results. At this time, no approach has been widely adopted to address the problem of multiple D-dimer assays, with different levels of technical complexity and different reference ranges. If a clinical laboratory also offers as part of a DIC panel, assays for FDP by a variety of methodologies, the confusion for physicians with regard to test selection and result interpretation for DIC is even greater.

Case with Error

A 25-year-old woman presents in the emergency room with shortness of breath after an 8-hour plane flight. To assess for the possibility of a pulmonary embolism in this patient considered to be of low probability for thrombosis, a D-dimer assay is requested at 4 PM. The laboratory that performs the D-dimer uses a highly sensitive enzyme-linked immunoassay for D-dimer until 4:30 PM, and then reverts to a less sensitive latex agglutination method for D-dimer measurement. The sample arrives in the laboratory after 4:30 PM, and as a result, a latex agglutination method is performed. The test is negative, but because of the insensitivity of the assay, the patient is further evaluated with a spiral CT scan. The time spent in the emergency room from presentation to discharge was 7 hours.

Explanation and Consequences

A negative result using the sensitive enzyme-linked D-dimer test in a patient with a low probability for pulmonary embolism would have provided a much more convincing reason to send the patient home without further evaluation. The poor sensitivity for pulmonary embolism of the latex agglutination test led to the need for imaging studies.

STANDARDS OF CARE

▦ The platelet count, the D-dimer, and the PT, with the possible addition of serial fibrinogen testing and a review of a peripheral blood smear, represent an acceptable and widely used group of tests to establish or rule out a diagnosis of DIC.

▦ Standard liver function tests may be useful to determine if DIC, liver disease, or both are present.

▦ Compensated DIC should be considered in patients who have a chronic stimulus for DIC, but this diagnosis may only become apparent when the compensatory mechanisms fail.

▦ Unless there are other reasons to do so, treatment of the acute DIC patient who is not bleeding with blood products is not indicated.

▓ The continued use of large amounts of blood products in the treatment of the bleeding patient with DIC should be guided by the treatability of the underlying condition stimulating the development of DIC.

▓ Education of physicians using the clinical laboratory about the assays used for D-dimer and FDP, in particular how they should be used clinically and their diagnostic limitations, is necessary to allow physicians to correctly interpret the results from these assays.

9 Evaluation for a Congenital Hypercoagulable State

OVERVIEW

There are several major challenges associated with evaluating a patient for hypercoagulability. One challenge is the identification of appropriate tests for inclusion in the hypercoagulation evaluation. There are five commonly assessed inherited conditions that predispose to thrombosis: the factor V Leiden mutation, the prothrombin 20210 mutation, and deficiencies of protein C, protein S, and antithrombin. Another challenge is to decide which patients should be evaluated with tests for hypercoagulability. There is no consensus on which patients to test even within the United States, and there is substantially more variability when comparing hypercoagulability testing in the United States with hypercoagulation test ordering practices in other countries. Included below are widely recognized errors in test ordering and test result interpretation in the assessment of patients for a congenital hypercoagulable state. Other chapters in this book present information on errors in the evaluation for antiphospholipid antibodies and for HIT that are associated with hypercoagulable states.

TEST ORDERING MISTAKES

▶ Ordering protein C and protein S levels in patients being treated with warfarin. True baseline protein C and protein S levels can be determined reliably 2 weeks after discontinuation of warfarin therapy, assuming the patient is able to synthesize proteins at a normal rate in the liver.

Case with Error

A 42-year-old man who developed a deep vein thrombosis 1 month earlier and is currently taking 5 mg of warfarin daily presents for assessment of thrombotic risk. A hypercoagulation test panel was ordered, which includes assays for protein C and protein S.

Explanation and Consequences

Warfarin decreases the levels of protein C and protein S from their baseline values. Therefore, a low level of either one of these proteins that might have been present from birth and contributory to the deep vein thrombosis is obscured because treatment with warfarin will produce low levels of these two proteins. The tests for protein C and protein S should not have been performed when the patient was receiving warfarin, and instead, they should have been delayed until warfarin had been discontinued for 1 to 2 weeks.

▶ Ordering the clot-based activated protein C resistance assay while the patient has a lupus anticoagulant or is receiving argatroban and/or lepirudin. All of these will interfere with this assay. To assess for the presence of factor V Leiden in such cases, the genetic test for the mutation must be performed, and the clot-based test for activated protein C resistance must be omitted.

Case with Error

A 28-year-old woman with two fetal losses is being evaluated for thrombotic risk with a hypercoagulation test panel. It is known that the patient has a positive test for the lupus anticoagulant, and a prolonged PTT on that basis. The screening test for the factor V Leiden mutation is a PTT-based assay known as the activated protein C resistance test. The doctor is unaware of the interference introduced by the lupus anticoagulant into this test. The activated protein C resistance test result is positive. The doctor pursues the positive activated protein C resistance test result by ordering a genetic test for the factor V Leiden mutation.

Explanation and Consequences

The correct course of action is to omit the activated protein C resistance test. This is because it was already known that the patient had a lupus anticoagulant with a prolonged PTT, which would likely produce a false-positive test result for activated protein C resistance. Such patients should be evaluated for the factor V Leiden mutation with a genetic test only. In this case, the doctor prolonged the evaluation and performed an unnecessary test.

> ▶ Ordering standard clot-based assays for protein C, protein S, and antithrombin while the patient is receiving argatroban or lepirudin. These compounds do not interfere with chromogenic assays, such as the chromogenic assay for protein C. These assays can only be performed if the direct thrombin inhibitor is no longer present in the specimen.

Case with Error

A 57-year-old man exposed to heparin develops HIT with a large pulmonary embolism, and for that reason is being anticoagulated with argatroban. While on argatroban, his doctor performs an evaluation for hypercoagulability. The results for protein C, protein S, and antithrombin are all markedly abnormal. The doctor concludes that the patient has multiple abnormalities in the concentration of these natural anticoagulants that have contributed to the development of his pulmonary embolism.

Explanation and Consequences

In this case, the argatroban interfered with the clot-based assays that were performed to measure the three natural anticoagulants. To accurately assess for a congenital deficiency of protein C, protein S, and antithrombin, the patient must be tested after argatroban has been discontinued for at least 3 to 4 hours. Unnecessary testing with misleading results were the consequences of this error.

> ▶ Ordering an assay for antithrombin for a patient who has been treated with full-dose unfractionated heparin or low molecular weight heparin. With such therapy, antithrombin forms a complex with heparin or low molecular weight heparin that is cleared, resulting in a low level for antithrombin that is not indicative of a true baseline antithrombin level for the patient. The patient's baseline antithrombin can be determined reliably 1 week after discontinuation of heparin or low molecular weight heparin therapy, assuming the patient is able to synthesize proteins at a normal rate in the liver.

Case with Error

A patient with a large femoral vein thrombosis is being treated with intravenous unfractionated heparin at a therapeutic dose. The patient has been receiving this treatment for the past 7 days and is now being evaluated for hypercoagulability with a test panel that includes an assay for antithrombin. The results for all of the tests in the panel are normal, with the exception of the antithrombin that is low. The doctor concludes that the patient has suffered the venous thrombosis as a result of a congenital antithrombin deficiency.

Explanation and Consequences

Patients treated with unfractionated heparin and low molecular weight heparin, particularly when these compounds are given at therapeutic doses rather than prophylactic doses, form antithrombin complexes with unfractionated heparin or low molecular weight heparin. In this case, this process of complex formation and subsequent clearance of the complexes decreased the level of circulating antithrombin. It is not possible to make a diagnosis of congenital antithrombin deficiency in patients who are being treated with heparin or low molecular weight heparin or in those who have recently been discontinued from treatment with these compounds. In the case described above, the patient will unnecessarily carry an incorrect diagnosis that could lead to indefinite treatment with oral anticoagulants, an evaluation of family members for antithrombin deficiency, and a persistent concern about recurrent thrombosis.

> ▶ Confusing factor V with the factor V Leiden mutation. For patients who are bleeding and being evaluated for a factor V deficiency, the correct test is the factor V assay. For patients who have experienced thrombosis, the correct test is the factor V Leiden.

Case with Error

A patient with venous thrombosis is evaluated with the factor V assay. The result is normal, and the doctor concludes that the patient does not have the factor V Leiden mutation.

Explanation and Consequences

The assays for factor V and factor V Leiden are distinct. A normal value for factor V has no influence on the presence or absence of the factor V Leiden mutation.

▶ Confusing factor II (prothrombin) with the prothrombin 20210 mutation. For patients who are bleeding and being evaluated for a factor II deficiency, the correct test is the factor II or prothrombin assay. For patients who have experienced thrombosis and are being evaluated for thrombotic risk, the correct test is the prothrombin 20210 mutation.

Case with Error

A patient with venous thrombosis is evaluated with a factor II assay. The result for factor II is 105%, which is a normal value. The doctor concludes that the patient does not have the prothrombin 20210 mutation.

Explanation and Consequences

The prothrombin assay measures the amount of factor II, and the assay for the prothrombin mutation 20210 determines the presence or absence of an altered prothrombin gene that results in a predisposition to thrombosis.

▶ Ordering protein S total antigen instead of protein S free antigen to assess for adequacy of protein S. The protein S total antigen is rarely decreased, and the functional protein S value correlates to the protein S free antigen.

Case with Error

The doctor orders a protein S total antigen assay to evaluate a patient for hypercoagulability. The result of the test is normal. The doctor concludes that there is no deficiency of protein S that could predispose his patient to thrombosis.

Explanation and Consequences

The active portion of protein S is the fraction which is free, that is, not bound to another protein. If a patient has a normal amount of protein S, but it is largely bound to other proteins and not free, the patient may have a significant predisposition to thrombosis. This important clinical finding will be missed if the assay for total protein S antigen is performed rather than the assay for protein S free antigen.

▶ Ordering antigenic tests for protein C, protein S, and antithrombin as first-line assays to assess for deficiencies of these proteins. Functional assays should be the first-line tests, as some patients who have deficiencies in these proteins will have normal antigenic levels but low functional levels. Ordering antigenic tests initially could result in a failure to identify important functional deficiencies of these three proteins.

Case with Error

A doctor evaluates a patient who has experienced recurrent venous thrombosis for hypercoagulability, and the assays for protein C, protein S, and antithrombin that are selected are all antigenic rather than functional. It is unknown to the doctor, and thereby also to the patient, that the patient has a functional deficiency of protein C, with a normal result for antigenic protein C. Because the doctor did not perform functional tests for these three proteins first, and received normal results for the antigenic tests, she prematurely ruled out deficiencies of any of these natural anticoagulants.

Explanation and Consequences

This patient has a congenital protein C deficiency that represents a significant predisposition to thrombosis that has been overlooked. The patient and the doctor remain unaware of his true functional protein C deficiency, and therefore none of his family members are evaluated for this risk factor.

▶ Ordering the test for methylene tetrahydrofolate reductase (MTHFR) as a risk factor for thrombosis. There is no proven association between abnormal levels of this enzyme and risk for thrombosis. It was recently thought that an elevated homocysteine is the thrombotic risk factor rather than an alteration in the activity of this enzyme in the homocysteine metabolic pathway. Ultimately, however, homocysteine was also disregarded as a risk factor for thrombosis, at least for modestly elevated homocysteine values that occur with minor vitamin deficiencies and renal dysfunction.

Case with Error

A woman with multiple fetal losses is evaluated with an assay for MTHFR. Her homocysteine level is normal.

Explanation and Consequences

There is no association between any result for MTHFR and risk for thrombosis or fetal loss. Testing for MTHFR in this setting is unnecessary.

▶ Ordering only protein C, protein S, and antithrombin for the patient to be evaluated for a hypercoagulable state, and omitting the more recently discovered common hypercoagulable states produced by the factor V Leiden mutation and the prothrombin 20210 mutation.

Case with Error

A patient is being evaluated for hypercoagulability and the test panel includes assays for protein C, protein S, and antithrombin. The patient is Caucasian. A series of normal values for all three of these proteins leads the doctor to conclude that his patient does not have a hypercoagulable state.

Explanation and Consequences

Caucasian patients in particular have a high incidence of the factor V Leiden mutation and the prothrombin 20210 mutation. The assays for protein C, protein S, and antithrombin were introduced onto many automated coagulation instrument platforms before the factor V Leiden and the prothrombin mutation were discovered. Because assays for the three natural anticoagulants have long been available in many clinical laboratories, it is not uncommon for a doctor to order tests for protein C, protein S, and antithrombin and not include assays for the factor V Leiden mutation and the prothrombin 20210 mutation. The latter two mutations are far more likely to be identified in a thrombotic patient because they are of much higher incidence, especially in Caucasians.

RESULT INTERPRETATION MISTAKES

Concluding that a deficiency of protein C, protein S, and/or antithrombin produced by an acquired condition is associated with an increased thrombotic risk. For the vast majority of cases, it is the congenital deficiencies of these proteins that result in an increased thrombotic risk. For example, patients with liver disease may demonstrate low levels of protein C, protein S, and antithrombin because these proteins are made in the liver. These patients are, however, typically not at increased risk for thrombosis because liver disease is also associated with deficiencies of the coagulation factors necessary to produce clotting. Therefore, liver disease has an effect that is both prothrombotic and antithrombotic, and as a result, the deficiencies of protein C, protein S, and antithrombin in patients with liver disease are not generally associated with an increased risk for thrombosis. A relatively balanced risk between thrombosis and bleeding is also seen in the patient ingesting warfarin at therapeutic levels. These patients have a low protein C and a low protein S, but they also have low levels of factors II, VII, IX, and X. The same can also be said for the patient who is being treated with heparin, who experiences a reduced antithrombin level as a result of heparin therapy.

Case with Error

A 33-year-old pregnant woman presents to her obstetrician for a routine evaluation. She provides a history of shortness of breath during a previous pregnancy that was never attributed to a pulmonary embolism. The doctor performs a hypercoagulation test panel because of this history. The results of the test panel are all normal except for a low value for free protein S. The doctor concludes that the low protein S value is a risk factor for thrombosis and recommends termination of the pregnancy, which the patient wishes to carry to term, to prevent the development of a potentially lethal thrombosis.

Explanation and Consequences

All pregnant women experience a decrease in protein S activity with pregnancy. Pregnancy is a hypercoagulable state, but there are many changes during pregnancy, and the acquired protein S deficiency found in virtually all pregnancies does not represent an isolated risk factor for thrombosis. The consequences of this misdiagnosis are severe if the patient terminates a normal pregnancy that she wishes to carry to term.

A confusing situation arises for low protein S values associated with two acquired conditions—a high estrogen state and an acute-phase reaction. A low value for protein S is found in patients with increased estrogen, such as those who are pregnant or taking estrogen supplements in the form of oral contraceptives or estrogen replacement therapy. The protein S can also be low in patients experiencing an acute-phase reaction. The high estrogen state and the acute-phase reaction do represent prothrombotic conditions, but the thrombotic tendency is not exclusively associated with the low value for protein S. There are a variety of coagulation abnormalities produced by a high estrogen state or an acute-phase response that promote thrombosis. Therefore, a low protein S associated with pregnancy or estrogen supplementation or an acute-phase response is in itself not considered a single major risk factor for thrombosis.

Case with Error

A 24-year-old woman, who is taking oral contraceptives, experiencing shortness of breath is evaluated for pulmonary embolism. The D-dimer result is borderline, and she is further evaluated for hypercoagulability. The only abnormality among the tests for hypercoagulability is a low protein S activity. The doctor incorrectly makes a diagnosis of a congenital deficiency of protein S, which predisposes to thrombosis.

Explanation and Consequences

Oral contraceptives and hormone replacement therapy result in a lowering of the protein S activity. It is important to understand that the low protein S in this young woman taking oral contraceptives does not represent a congenital deficiency of this protein and a predisposition to thrombosis. In this case, the patient acquired an incorrect diagnosis and raised concern within her family of a genetic predisposition to thrombosis. There is a danger for future errors in anticoagulation because of this diagnostic mistake.

> ▶ Failing to understand that the reference ranges for protein C, protein S, and antithrombin in children are different from the corresponding reference ranges for these factors in adults. Protein C is especially late in normalizing to the adult reference range and values for children below the age of 8 or 9 years are not correctly assessed using the adult reference range. Because of this, children should be evaluated for protein C, protein S, and antithrombin using an appropriate age-adjusted reference range for each factor.

Case with Error

A 2-year-old child has a protein C value that is well below the listed reference range for the clinical laboratory performing the protein C assay. The doctor mistakenly concludes that the child has a protein C deficiency, which predisposes to thrombosis.

Explanation and Consequences

Age-adjusted reference ranges are especially important in the determination of deficiencies of protein C, protein S, and antithrombin. In this case, a child is inappropriately identified as congenitally deficient in protein C, which can lead to inappropriate anticoagulation in the future and unnecessary testing of the patient and the patient's first-degree relatives.

CONTROVERSY

Ordering protein C, protein S, and antithrombin in patients who are actively clotting. Active clotting is associated with consumption of these factors, and therefore, deficiencies observed during this time do not reflect the patient's true baseline levels of these natural anticoagulant proteins. It is important to not misdiagnose a patient as congenitally deficient in protein C, protein S, or antithrombin during a period of active clotting. Many such patients show only a mild decrease in these three proteins, such that diagnosis of a deficiency state, if one exists, is still usually possible during clot formation. These patients typically increase their levels of these proteins to their baseline values, whatever they are, within a day or two after an acute thrombotic event, assuming normal liver function to permit protein synthesis at a normal rate. Some physicians recommend tests for these proteins only after an acute thrombotic event has clearly subsided, and often when the patient is no longer in the hospital. Other physicians recommend immediate testing so that the patient is sure to be evaluated for a hypercoagulable state. In addition, collection of a blood sample before a patient with venous thrombosis receives anticoagulants provides laboratory values for protein C, protein S, and antithrombin that are not confounded by anticoagulant therapy.

Considering the homocysteine value to assess for thrombotic risk. Modest elevations of homocysteine associated with vitamin deficiencies or renal dysfunction do not appear to be associated with an increased thrombotic risk. However, it has not been established whether very significantly elevated homocysteine values, for example, above 30 μmol/L are associated with thrombotic risk. Patients with very high homocysteine levels may have an inherited defect in homocysteine metabolism. One congenital disorder associated with markedly elevated homocysteine levels is a deficiency of the enzyme cystathionine beta-synthase.

Ordering hypercoagulation studies prior to making a decision about the use of oral contraceptives. The combination of oral contraceptives and a genetic deficiency associated with thrombosis greatly increases the risk of a clotting event. For that reason, some argue that a hypercoagulation panel should be performed before prescribing oral contraceptives. The cost to the health care system from evaluating women with a negative personal and family thrombotic history with hypercoagulation studies is not insignificant, and this is the principal argument for not performing the tests. At a minimum, however, there is wide agreement that a careful personal history and family history for thrombosis should be taken before providing any recommendation for oral contraceptive use.

STANDARDS OF CARE

■ Order tests for activated protein C resistance, protein C, protein S, and antithrombin in the absence of interfering factors, commonly anticoagulants, which make the results of these tests uninterpretable and not representative of the patient's true baseline values.

■ Order functional rather than antigenic tests for protein C, protein S, and antithrombin as first-line tests for assessment of hypercoagulability.

■ Avoid the use of MTHFR as a test for thrombotic risk, and do not conclude that modest elevations in homocysteine represent a risk for thrombosis.

■ Identify the factor V Leiden mutation and the prothrombin 20210 mutation and congenital deficiencies of protein C, protein S, and antithrombin as risks for thrombosis; with the understanding that acquired deficiencies of protein C, protein S, and antithrombin are unlikely to represent risks for thrombosis because these deficiencies typically occur at the same time when there is an increased risk for bleeding.

■ Age-adjusted reference ranges must be used in the assessment of children for deficiencies of protein C, protein S, and antithrombin.

10 Evaluation for Antiphospholipid Antibodies

OVERVIEW

For patients with thrombotic disorders, tests for antiphospholipid antibodies are commonly performed. Antiphospholipid antibodies represent a large category of antibodies directed at the protein beta-2 glycoprotein I. The function of this protein and its relationship to thrombosis remain to be fully elucidated, although much progress is being made. Antibodies to beta-2 glycoprotein I can be measured in a clot-based assay known as the lupus anticoagulant test. In addition, such antibodies can be detected in enzyme-linked immunoassay tests for anticardiolipin antibodies and for anti–beta-2 glycoprotein I antibodies, and these may be specific to domain 1 of the beta-2 glycoprotein I protein. There is another increasingly recognized antiphospholipid antibody that recognizes factor II (prothrombin), which is bound to the negatively charged phospholipid known as phosphatidylserine. There is substantial confusion among practitioners regarding which antiphospholipid antibody tests should be ordered and how the results for these tests should be interpreted. In general, the more the antiphospholipid antibody tests that are positive, and the higher the test results are above the upper limit of normal, the greater is the risk for a thrombotic event.

TEST ORDERING MISTAKES

▶ Failing to order enough tests to assess for antiphospholipid antibodies. There is a growing consensus that, among the different antiphospholipid antibody tests, the lupus anticoagulant test is the one most associated with thrombotic risk. However, some patients have a negative test for the lupus anticoagulant, while testing positive for anticardiolipin antibodies or anti–beta-2 glycoprotein I antibodies. For this reason, if a patient is being evaluated for thrombotic risk with tests for antiphospholipid antibodies, tests for the lupus anticoagulant as well as tests for anticardiolipin or anti–beta-2 glycoprotein I antibodies should be performed to perform a thorough evaluation for the presence of an antiphospholipid antibody.

Case with Error

A 32-year-old woman who has suffered three pregnancy losses before the 10th week is evaluated with the lupus anticoagulant to assess for the presence of antiphospholipid antibody syndrome. A test for the lupus anticoagulant is negative. No further testing to diagnose antiphospholipid antibody syndrome is performed, and the doctor concludes that she does not suffer from this syndrome.

Explanation and Consequences

This patient was found to have highly elevated values for IgG and IgM anticardiolipin antibodies. Failure to make the diagnosis of antiphospholipid antibody syndrome in this patient decreased the likelihood that the patient would be offered anticoagulant therapy to try to carry a future pregnancy to term.

▶ Ordering too many antiphospholipid antibody tests. There are many tests commercially available for the lupus anticoagulant. A screening test and a confirmatory test that are phospholipid dependent have long been considered adequate to assess a patient or the lupus anticoagulant. There are at least five other commercially available tests for the lupus anticoagulant. For anticardiolipin antibodies, it is possible to test for IgG, IgM, and IgA antibodies. The same three antibody classes can also be measured for anti–beta-2 glycoprotein I antibodies. There are also commercially available tests for anti-prothrombin and antiphosphatidylserine antibodies (IgG, IgM, and IgA). A common practice is to quantify only IgG and IgM antibodies when assessing a patient for anticardiolipin antibodies or anti–beta-2 glycoprotein I antibodies. Thus, one can perform more than a dozen different tests to search for antiphospholipid antibodies, but performing these tests until one is found to be positive is considered inappropriate.

Case with Error

A 22-year-old woman with signs and symptoms consistent with an autoimmune disorder is evaluated with antiphospholipid antibody tests. The screening test for the lupus anticoagulant, anticardiolipin antibodies (IgG and IgM), and anti–beta-2 glycoprotein I antibodies (IgG and IgM) are all negative. In an attempt to identify an antiphospholipid antibody in this patient, three different tests for the lupus anticoagulant and IgG, IgM, and IgA anti-prothrombin antibodies are then requested. The IgA test for anti-prothrombin antibodies is the only positive test result obtained.

Explanation and Consequences

There is no universal standard for the appropriate number of antiphospholipid antibody tests to be performed when searching for such an antibody. However, most experts would consider an evaluation like the one described in this case to represent excessive testing. When one uncommonly performed antiphospholipid antibody test is positive, among many different negative tests for the antibody, the clinical significance of a lone positive test for antiphospholipid antibody syndrome, thrombotic risk, or fetal loss is particularly uncertain.

> ▶ Not performing a confirmatory phospholipid-dependent test for the lupus anticoagulant following a positive screening test. Screening tests for the lupus anticoagulant based upon the PTT have many interferences that generate false-positive test results. For this reason, a confirmatory phospholipid-dependent assay for the lupus anticoagulant is essential to accurately determine whether the patient has a lupus anticoagulant.

Case with Error

A 78-year-old man receiving intravenous unfractionated heparin is awaiting coronary artery bypass grafting. As part of an evaluation for thrombotic risk, the patient is tested for a lupus anticoagulant with the standard PTT-based screening test. The test result is positive. No confirmatory phospholipid-dependent assay for the lupus anticoagulant is performed, and the doctor concludes at this point in the evaluation that the patient has a lupus anticoagulant. In addition, no information is provided to the laboratory to indicate that the patient is receiving intravenous heparin at the time the sample is collected for the lupus anticoagulant test.

Explanation and Consequences

Unfractionated heparin can prolong the PTT, and on that basis, will produce a false-positive test for the lupus anticoagulant in the commonly used PTT-based screening test. If the clinical laboratory were made aware of the presence of heparin, the patient sample could have been processed to remove the heparin before analysis for the lupus anticoagulant, in both screening and confirmatory tests. In this case, the presence of heparin as an interfering substance prevented the determination of the true lupus anticoagulant status. In addition, the false-positive result for this patient may have led to a misleading conclusion that the patient is predisposed to thrombosis because of the presence of a lupus anticoagulant.

RESULT INTERPRETATION MISTAKES

▶ Concluding that the presence of a lupus anticoagulant is an indication that the patient has the disease systemic lupus erythematosus or that the patient has an anticoagulant. Unfortunately, the lupus anticoagulant was first found in two women with lupus and was named as a result of this association. Many healthy asymptomatic individuals and many patients with disorders other than autoimmune diseases are found to have a lupus anticoagulant. Also unfortunately, the lupus anticoagulant was found to prolong the time for clot formation in laboratory coagulation tests. Paradoxically, in vivo, the presence of the lupus anticoagulant itself does not confer a bleeding risk, but may confer a thrombotic risk. Thus, both "lupus" and "anticoagulant" are misleading terms.

Case with Error

The doctor informs a young adult female patient that she has a lupus anticoagulant. No further explanation is provided. The doctor fails to provide additional information because of his own limited knowledge about the clinical significance of a lupus anticoagulant.

Explanation and Consequences

The patient hears only the word "lupus" and concludes that she carries a diagnosis of systemic lupus erythematosus. She fails to understand that she does not have a serious autoimmune disorder, and also does not appreciate the connection of the lupus anticoagulant to an increased predisposition for a thrombosis and complications of pregnancy.

▶ Confusing a lupus anticoagulant for a factor VIII inhibitor and confusing a factor VIII inhibitor for a lupus anticoagulant. It is often difficult to conclusively demonstrate that a patient has one of these entities but not the other. Clinically however, it is extremely important to do so, because patients with a factor VIII inhibitor may have catastrophic bleeding, and patients with the lupus anticoagulant may develop serious thrombosis. As a result, the treatment for these two entities is completely the opposite. The challenge arises because the presence of a factor VIII inhibitor can produce a false-positive test for the lupus anticoagulant; and the presence of a lupus anticoagulant can result in a low factor VIII level in the test for coagulation factor VIII in the laboratory. One way to attempt to differentiate a lupus anticoagulant from a factor VIII inhibitor is to perform assays for coagulation factors VIII, IX, XI, and XII. These are all PTT-related coagulation factor assays, and as noted previously, the lupus anticoagulant in a vast majority of cases prolongs the PTT and not the PT. As noted in Chapter 7 on PT, PTT, and coagulation factors, the assays for coagulation factors should be performed at multiple plasma dilutions to assess for the presence of a coagulation factor inhibitor. When a lupus anticoagulant is present, an inhibitor is detected in more than one of the four PTT-related coagulation factor assays, and the factors that are lowered are decreased approximately to the same extent by this inhibitor. On the other hand, factor VIII inhibitors typically result in a markedly low value only for factor VIII, with higher values for factors IX, XI, and XII. Some patients with a factor VIII inhibitor will have a negative test for a lupus anticoagulant. When this situation arises, it is much easier to differentiate the patient with a factor VIII inhibitor from one with the lupus anticoagulant.

Case with Error

An 82-year-old man presents with a prolonged PTT in a preoperative evaluation. He was found to have a prolonged PTT on multiple occasions over the past 20 years. He was told that he has a factor VIII inhibitor when his prolonged PTT was first noticed 20 years ago. Before surgery at that time, he was given factor VIII concentrate, and there was no excess bleeding with the procedure. The interpretation by the surgeon at that time was that the patient must have had a factor VIII inhibitor, and the bleeding was prevented by the administration of factor VIII concentrate before surgery. The surgeon did not consider that a factor VIII inhibitor may not have been present and that treatment with factor VIII concentrate was unnecessary. A review of the evaluation for the prolonged PTT from 20 years ago reveals that the patient had a prolonged PTT that failed to correct in a PTT mixing study at any time point after mixing his plasma with normal plasma. In addition, the patient had evidence for the presence of an inhibitor that similarly affected factor VIII as well as the other PTT-related factors (IX, XI, and XII). These results are much more consistent with the presence of a lupus anticoagulant, rather than with a factor VIII inhibitor.

Explanation and Consequences

The danger of receiving factor VIII concentrate in the early 1980s was that the product at that time was often contaminated with HIV and hepatitis C. For two decades this patient carried a misdiagnosis that resulted on at least one occasion with his receiving a pooled blood product (factor VIII concentrate) from several donors. Fortunately for this patient, he did not develop HIV or hepatitis C.

CONTROVERSY

▶ It is still not well established whether it is advisable to evaluate a patient for antiphospholipid antibodies using both anticardiolipin antibody tests and anti–beta-2 glycoprotein I antibody tests. These are both enzyme-linked immunoassay tests in which an antibody from the patient binds to the protein beta-2 glycoprotein I. The assays are constructed somewhat differently, and for that reason there is a concern that an antibody might be detected using one assay but not the other. Generally speaking, if there is a high suspicion for an antiphospholipid antibody in a patient with a negative test for the lupus anticoagulant, tests for anticardiolipin antibodies and anti–beta-2 glycoprotein I antibodies might both be ordered in an effort to detect antiphospholipid antibodies. Enthusiasm is decreasing at the present time for the use of anticardiolipin antibody tests.

STANDARDS OF CARE

▨ The assessment of a patient for the presence of antiphospholipid antibodies should include a correctly performed screening that and a phospholipid-dependent lupus anticoagulant test if the screening test is positive, as well as assays for IgG and IgM anticardiolipin or anti–beta-2 glycoprotein I antibodies.

▨ A lupus anticoagulant must be clearly differentiated from a factor VIII inhibitor.

▨ Patients with a lupus anticoagulant alone should not be presumed to have the disease lupus or to suffer from a bleeding predisposition.

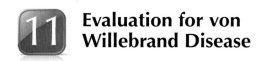

11 Evaluation for von Willebrand Disease

OVERVIEW

The diagnosis of von Willebrand disease is typically initiated with a request for tests for von Willebrand factor antigen, ristocetin cofactor, and factor VIII. Patients can significantly elevate their values for these assays above their true baseline levels with even a mild stimulation of the acute-phase response. As a result, many patients who have a von Willebrand factor level or ristocetin cofactor level consistent with von Willebrand disease are misdiagnosed as being free from the disease because their values were elevated as part of the acute-phase response at the time they were studied. Repeat testing in the absence of all stimuli to the acute-phase response is absolutely essential, and this may require several evaluations of the patient to confidently determine whether a patient has von Willebrand disease.

TEST ORDERING MISTAKES

> ▶ Ordering a von Willebrand multimer analysis to further evaluate a patient whose results for von Willebrand factor antigen, ristocetin cofactor, and factor VIII strongly indicate the presence of type 1 von Willebrand disease. Most patients with von Willebrand disease have type 1. Therefore, unless there is a reason from the results of the initial tests for von Willebrand factor, ristocetin cofactor, and factor VIII to suspect a von Willebrand type other than type 1, it is unnecessary to test for von Willebrand multimers.

Case with Error

A patient with a mild history of bleeding is evaluated for von Willebrand disease. The results of the tests for von Willebrand factor antigen, ristocetin cofactor, and factor VIII are 36%, 39%, and 38%, respectively. The doctor then orders a test for von Willebrand multimers to further evaluate the patient for the type of von Willebrand disease that appears to be present.

Explanation and Consequences

This is a classic case of type 1 von Willebrand disease. The evaluation for von Willebrand multimers to establish this case as type 1 is considered by most experts to be unnecessary. The cost of testing for von Willebrand multimers is significant.

Not ordering a complete von Willebrand panel, which minimally consists of tests for von Willebrand factor antigen and ristocetin cofactor. The inclusion of factor VIII is often informative and considered necessary by many in the initial screening for von Willebrand disease. The test for ristocetin cofactor shows much analytical variability and is time consuming. Because of this, for cases requiring a rapid indication of the presence or absence of von Willebrand disease, a von Willebrand factor antigen test may be useful as an initial assessment of the disease. However, final conclusions regarding a diagnosis of von Willebrand disease should be made using the results from von Willebrand factor antigen and ristocetin cofactor, and factor VIII if it is performed.

Case with Error

A clinical laboratory in a 200-bed community hospital does not perform tests for von Willebrand disease. A patient evaluated in this hospital for von Willebrand disease has a blood sample collected and sent to an outside laboratory that performs testing for the disease. To minimize the cost of this analysis, a single test for ristocetin cofactor is requested. The result of this assay is 45% of normal.

Explanation and Consequences

The diagnosis of von Willebrand disease is often challenging, and in this case, it is even more challenging because only one of the commonly used tests in a von Willebrand panel was performed. Because of this, the likelihood for a misdiagnosis of the disease is greatly increased for this patient. There is significant variability in the results for assays in the von Willebrand panel. One contributory factor is that von Willebrand factor increases significantly as part of the acute-phase response. Another contributory factor is that the ristocetin cofactor assay in particular has a high analytical variability.

RESULT INTERPRETATION MISTAKES

▶Failing to understand that von Willebrand factor, as measured by von Willebrand factor antigen and as ristocetin cofactor, increases in the presence of an acute-phase response. Therefore, patients suffering from infections, patients who have been injured, and those affected by other stimuli of the acute-phase response, can experience an increase of 2- to 3-fold over baseline of both von Willebrand factor antigen and ristocetin cofactor. This can result in the incorrect conclusion that a patient with a von Willebrand factor baseline level well below normal is completely free of von Willebrand disease.

Case with Error

A 6-month-old child with undiagnosed von Willebrand disease falls from a bed onto a hardwood floor and is evaluated shortly after the injury with tests for this disease because of the presence of a subdural hematoma and a history of excessive bruising provided by the parents. The results for the von Willebrand panel are all within the reference range established by the clinical laboratory performing the tests. The doctor concludes that the child does not suffer from von Willebrand disease.

Explanation and Consequences

Tragic consequence can follow from an incorrect conclusion that a patient does not have von Willebrand disease when the testing for this disorder is performed during an acute-phase response, and the patient is not reevaluated after the acute-phase response is over. The failure to establish the true baseline levels of von Willebrand factor and ristocetin cofactor in bleeding children, such as the one in this case, by retesting after an acute-phase response is over has resulted in accusations of innocent fathers of child abuse when, in fact, the children suffered from undiagnosed von Willebrand disease, and a minor injury led to major bleeding.

> ▶ Failing to understand that the reference range for von Willebrand factor antigen in children less than 6 months of age is higher than the reference range for this protein in individuals older than 6 months. Therefore, a value that might be normal for someone older than 6 months could be low for a child younger than 6 months. Because of this, children should be evaluated for von Willebrand disease using an appropriate age-adjusted reference range.

Case with Error

A 1-month-old baby boy is evaluated for von Willebrand disease with a test for von Willebrand factor antigen because of a family history of this disorder and the presence of bruises. The result of the test is 55% of normal. This is considered by the doctor to be within the reference range established by the laboratory. The laboratory does not have an age-adjusted reference range for von Willebrand factor.

Explanation and Consequences

A value of 50% of normal for von Willebrand factor in an adult is less suggestive of a diagnosis of von Willebrand disease than it is for a child under the age of 6 months. Children in this age group have a reference range that is higher than the reference range for adults for von Willebrand factor. A misinterpretation by the doctor about the child in this case may remove von Willebrand disease from further consideration to explain any future bleeding episodes, and thereby, lead to inappropriate treatment.

CONTROVERSY

▶ The threshold for von Willebrand factor antigen and ristocetin cofactor, below which a diagnosis of von Willebrand disease is rendered, remains controversial. The trend has been to use increasingly lower thresholds to establish the diagnosis of this disease. Guidelines driven by opinion experts are emerging, but there is significant controversy about them because so many patients above a threshold recommended for diagnosis of von Willebrand disease clearly have a bleeding disorder that is decreased by elevation of von Willebrand factor with DDAVP. These patients do not formally qualify for a diagnosis.

A major confounding variable in the establishment of a reference range for von Willebrand disease using von Willebrand factor or ristocetin cofactor is that the blood type of the patient greatly influences the amount of von Willebrand factor. Patients with blood group O have approximately 74% of the normal amount of von Willebrand factor, and patients with type AB blood have as much as 125% of the normal amount of von Willebrand factor. Patients with type A and type B have mean values between 74% and 125%, with type B patients being higher than patients with type A. The general consensus at this point appears to consider bleeding risk based upon the absolute amount of von Willebrand factor and ristocetin cofactor, independent of the blood type. As a result, patients with type O blood require a modest decrease in von Willebrand factor or ristocetin cofactor from their mean value of 74% to receive a diagnosis of von Willebrand disease. This is in contrast to the patient with type AB blood who requires a major decrease from 125% to achieve a diagnosis of von Willebrand disease.

STANDARDS OF CARE

▤ The appropriate testing to initially evaluate a patient for von Willebrand disease includes von Willebrand factor antigen and ristocetin cofactor minimally, with factor VIII commonly included in the initial testing.

▤ Normal values for von Willebrand factor antigen and ristocetin cofactor in a bleeding patient suspected of von Willebrand disease should be considered as possibly elevated from an acute-phase stimulus. Repeat testing for the disease should be performed to confirm or deny the presence of this disorder if there is reason to be suspicious of an acute phase response.

▤ Despite variations in von Willebrand factor antigen and ristocetin cofactor with blood type, the threshold for diagnosis of von Willebrand disease is commonly made without consideration of the patient's blood type.

▤ Age-adjusted reference ranges must be used in the diagnosis of von Willebrand disease.

12 Evaluation for a Coagulation Factor VIII Inhibitor

OVERVIEW

The presence of a factor VIII inhibitor can lead to major bleeding. The identification of the inhibitor, which requires its differentiation from the lupus anticoagulant, and its subsequent quantitation in Bethesda units is essential to identify and correctly manage the patient with a factor VIII inhibitor. The test for the factor VIII inhibitor is one of the most complex assays performed in the clinical laboratory. It should be performed only in cases in which there is significant evidence from a PTT mixing study and a factor VIII assay (as detailed below) that a factor VIII inhibitor is present. The treatment options for a factor VIII inhibitor are all extremely expensive (cases have been reported in which hundreds of thousands of dollars have been spent on a single patient), and they all present a measurable thrombotic risk. Thus, it is possible to convert a bleeding patient with a factor VIII inhibitor into one with a catastrophic thrombosis. The treatment selected is significantly influenced by the Bethesda unit value. Therefore, the accurate measurement of antibodies to factor VIII is important because it guides the appropriate use of highly expensive and potentially thrombotic compounds.

TEST ORDERING MISTAKES

▶Requesting quantitation of the antibody to factor VIII in Bethesda units when there is no evidence from the PTT mixing study or the factor VIII level to suspect an antibody to factor VIII. The PTT mixing study shows a classic response in patients with a factor VIII inhibitor. The PTT of the mixed plasma initially corrects into the reference range or shortens significantly toward normal, but as the mixed plasma is allowed to incubate at 37°C for up to 1 to 2 hours, the PTT increases. The antibody to factor VIII requires time in the mixed plasma to bind and neutralize the factor VIII, and thereby produce this result in the mixing study (initial correction which fades) suggestive of a factor VIII inhibitor. The PTT increase over the incubation time in the mixing study with normal plasma is approximately reflective of the strength of the inhibitor in Bethesda units.

Case with Error

A 78-year-old man presents with persistent hematuria over the past month. The doctor identifies a prolongation of the PTT to 65 seconds. A PTT mixing study that is performed fails to correct into the normal range at any time point. This result is consistent with the presence of a lupus anticoagulant. The doctor requests an assay to quantitate the amount of antibody to factor VIII and never requests an assay for the lupus anticoagulant. This request is made in the absence of a PTT mixing study result consistent with the presence of a factor VIII inhibitor or a low factor VIII level.

Explanation and Consequences

In this case, the doctor was intent on identifying an explanation for bleeding. This raised the possibility of a factor VIII inhibitor because it is associated with bleeding, and it can spontaneously arise in older patients. This is unlike the lupus anticoagulant which is not associated with bleeding. The PTT mixing study and the factor VIII level ruled out a factor VIII inhibitor as a possible explanation for the patient's hematuria. The negative consequence of the doctor's decision is the unnecessary performance of an extremely time-consuming and expensive laboratory test to quantify the number of Bethesda units of anti-factor VIII antibody.

RESULT INTERPRETATION MISTAKES

> ▶ Incorrectly identifying a lupus anticoagulant, present in 3% to 5% of healthy individuals, as a much rarer factor VIII inhibitor, and conversely mistaking a rare factor VIII inhibitor as a lupus anticoagulant. This situation is presented in significant detail as the second concept in Chapter 10 on antiphospholipid antibodies under the "Result Interpretation Mistakes" section.

Case with Error

A 70-year-old man with a new onset of easy bruising is found to have an elevated PTT. Further evaluation of the PTT prolongation with a test for the lupus anticoagulant is positive. The doctor concludes that the patient has an elevated PTT on the basis of a lupus anticoagulant. No further testing is performed.

Explanation and Consequences

A PTT mixing study at this point would be very useful to differentiate a lupus anticoagulant from a factor VIII inhibitor. In addition, an assay for factor VIII that is essentially normal at the highest plasma dilution tested makes a factor VIII inhibitor in this case extremely unlikely. A factor VIII inhibitor will reduce the level of factor VIII in the circulation and on that basis prolong the PTT. The inhibitory action of this antibody will also produce a false-positive test in a commonly used PTT-based lupus anticoagulant assay. A factor VIII inhibitor must be promptly identified, quantified, and appropriately treated to prevent major bleeding. This patient already has evidence of bleeding, providing a clue that the underlying problem is a factor VIII inhibitor rather than a lupus anticoagulant. The testing strategy described above indicates how a factor VIII inhibitor and a lupus anticoagulant are differentiated.

▶ Treating a patient with a factor VIII inhibitor with factor VIII concentrate when the Bethesda unit level indicates that there is too much anti-factor VIII antibody for the concentrate to be effective. Bethesda unit values above 4 to 10 (published studies show different thresholds within this range) should indicate a need to use a product other than factor VIII concentrate to treat bleeding. Commonly used treatments for such patients include recombinant factor VIIa and prothrombin complex concentrates. It is useful to note that in most patients with a factor VIII inhibitor, each additional Bethesda unit decreases the amount of factor VIII by approximately 50%. Therefore, only 7 Bethesda units can decrease a value of 100% factor VIII to: 50% (1)–25% (2)–12.5% (3)–6.25% (4)–3.12% (5)–1.66% (6)–0.8% (7). Many patients with factor VIII inhibitors have values above 7 Bethesda units.

Case with Error Averted

A 58-year-old woman presents with a mass in her abdomen which requires the performance of a hysterectomy. Before surgery, she is found to have a prolonged PTT. Further evaluation reveals that she has an anti-factor VIII antibody with a Bethesda unit titer of 260 units. The anesthesiologist requests factor VIII concentrate to be given to this patient before surgery. Consultation with a doctor specializing in hemostasis and thrombosis results in withdrawal of the request for this product.

Explanation and Consequences

The concentration of anti-factor VIII antibody in the circulation of this patient would overwhelm any amount of factor VIII concentrate, and thereby make the factor VIII concentrate ineffective in preventing excess bleeding with surgery. More effective treatment options for patients like this one include the use of recombinant factor VIIa or prothrombin complex concentrates.

STANDARDS OF CARE

▓ The highly complex and expensive test for quantitation of the antibody to factor VIII in Bethesda units should not be ordered unless there is evidence from the PTT mixing study or the factor VIII level to suspect an antibody to factor VIII.

▓ A factor VIII inhibitor and a lupus anticoagulant should be clearly differentiated, using the appropriate laboratory tests.

▓ The treatment option selected for a patient with a factor VIII inhibitor should be appropriate for the number of Bethesda units quantitated in the assay.

13 Evaluation for Thrombocytopenia That Is Not Associated with Heparin Exposure

OVERVIEW

Errors associated with spuriously high or low platelet counts are commonly observed in the clinical laboratory. One of the most common causes of a spuriously low platelet count results from a problem of insufficient mixing at the time of blood collection. This can occur when the blood in the tube is not gently agitated back and forth several times to mix the dried EDTA anticoagulant in the tube with the blood. In some cases, the laboratory can identify a platelet count as spurious by further analysis before it is reported. However, in other situations, the physician needs to have a high level of suspicion that a platelet count, which is significantly different from recent platelet counts on the same patient, is spurious, to avoid a misdiagnosis. Laboratory testing can be performed to identify a limited number of causes for a true thrombocytopenia. Such laboratory tests, however, are often present only in large clinical laboratories. Examples of these assays are the ADAMTS 13 assays for thrombotic thrombocytopenic purpura (TTP) and drug-induced thrombocytopenia assays for heparin (see Chapter 6 on HIT) and compounds other than heparin.

TEST ORDERING MISTAKES

▶ Not considering a medication recently initiated for a patient as a cause for thrombocytopenia. There are many medications that are associated with the development of thrombocytopenia. Although uncommonly performed, assays are available to assess for drug-induced thrombocytopenia for compounds other than heparin. A positive test in such an assay provides at least a tentative diagnosis for drug-induced thrombocytopenia associated with that drug. A confirmed diagnosis can be established if the platelet count recovers after discontinuation of the suspected medication.

Case with Error

A 31-year-old man is treated with sulfonamides, and over the course of the next 2 weeks notices the development of petechiae. He presents to his doctor who notices a low platelet count. The doctor fails to consider drug-induced thrombocytopenia associated with sulfonamides in the differential diagnosis.

Explanation and Consequences

The substantial attention directed toward heparin as a cause of drug-induced thrombocytopenia has obscured to some extent the fact that other drugs that can produce thrombocytopenia. This case describes an example with sulfonamides, which can induce drug-induced thrombocytopenia.

> ▶ Ordering a test for antiplatelet antibodies by flow cytometry or other method in the diagnostic evaluation for immune thrombocytopenia (ITP). Although such testing is available, it has minimal clinical utility in this setting.

Case with Error

A 24-year-old woman presents with petechiae of recent onset. Further evaluation leads to a clinical diagnosis of ITP. The doctor wishes to confirm the diagnosis by demonstrating the presence of a platelet-associated antibody. A blood sample is collected from the patient and sent to an outside laboratory to determine the amount of platelet-associated antibody by flow cytometry.

Explanation and Consequences

Though a platelet-associated antibody is associated with the pathogenesis of this disease, testing for the presence of such an antibody is not confirmatory for a diagnosis of ITP. This error subjects the patient to an unnecessary blood collection and creates an unnecessary expense for a costly assay.

RESULT INTERPRETATION MISTAKES

▶ Overlooking platelet clumping induced by EDTA in a purple top Vacutainer containing EDTA as an anticoagulant. Such platelet clumping leads to a diagnosis of "pseudo-thrombocytopenia" because the platelet count is not decreased in the patient, only in the blood sample. A review of a blood smear made with a sample of whole blood from such a patient would reveal platelet clumps to suggest a diagnosis of pseudo-thrombocytopenia. Collection of blood for a platelet count into a tube with citrate and no EDTA confirms the diagnosis if the platelet count is normal.

Case with Error

A 45-year-old woman presents for a routine annual evaluation. A complete blood count is performed, and the platelet count is noted to be markedly reduced. The patient shows no signs of bleeding and has previously been found to have a normal platelet count. An extensive evaluation is planned to determine the cause of the thrombocytopenia.

Explanation and Consequences

A repeat platelet count should be performed to assess the reproducibility of the low platelet count. One diagnostic possibility for any sample showing a low platelet count is the unusual anomaly whereby EDTA in the blood collection tube promotes the clumping of platelets before analysis. The platelet clumps are not recognized as platelets by the automated blood cell counter. A peripheral blood smear made from this sample reveals many large platelet aggregates. A repeat platelet count using a sample collected in a different anticoagulant is normal. Until the artifact was identified, the patient and her family were very concerned about the possibility of a much more serious explanation for the thrombocytopenia.

▶ Failing to review and act upon an extremely low platelet count in a timely fashion. Platelet counts that are especially low, particularly those less than 10 000 per microliter, can be associated with spontaneous bleeding and produce significantly adverse clinical outcomes. A very low platelet count is typically regarded as a critical value requiring immediate notification of a caregiver.

Case with Error

A platelet count of 9000 per microliter is identified in a 6-year-old boy who has recently experienced an upper respiratory tract infection. The doctor fails to consider a diagnosis of acute ITP in this patient and takes no action to address the low platelet count.

Explanation and Consequences

Although nearly all children who develop acute ITP spontaneously normalize their platelet count without treatment, the danger of a serious bleed exists, when the platelet count is particularly low. At a minimum, recognition of this low platelet count would be important to minimize the likelihood of even minor trauma while the platelet count is especially low.

▶ Failing to recognize a low platelet count as attributable to TTP as a possible diagnosis. TTP is a rare but life-threatening condition. If a patient suffering from TTP is treated by apheresis, the mortality from this disorder decreases dramatically. A constellation of laboratory and clinical findings provides a relative likelihood for a diagnosis of TTP. At the current time, assays for the enzyme activity (ADAMTS 13) deficient in patients with TTP are being performed in a limited number of clinical laboratories. Despite the low incidence of this disorder, the potentially devastating clinical consequences of a missed diagnosis of TTP and the expense and invasiveness of apheresis have all promoted the rapid development of ADAMTS 13 assays that can be performed without especially sophisticated laboratory equipment.

Case with Error

A hospitalized patient develops a clinical picture that could be consistent TTP or DIC. Apheresis is life saving if the diagnosis is TTP, but potentially dangerous if the diagnosis is DIC. There is no assay immediately available for ADAMTS 13 in the clinical laboratory of this hospital.

Explanation and Consequences

In this case, an error often occurs in the presence of good clinical judgment. Commonly, apheresis is performed in the absence of a firm diagnosis of TTP because failure to perform this procedure can lead to the death of the patient if TTP is present. As soon as the result is available for the ADAMTS 13 test for such a patient, a more informed diagnosis of TTP or DIC can be made, with a decision on the need for apheresis.

> ▶ Assuming that thrombocytopenia from all causes is effec-
> tively treated with transfusion of platelet concentrates. As
> noted in Chapter 6 on HIT, platelet transfusions given to patients
> with this disorder, for example, can result in thrombosis that is
> associated with significant morbidity and mortality.

In Chapter 6 on HIT, the second case in the "Result Interpretation
Mistakes" section describes an error associated with transfusion of
platelet concentrates in a patient with HIT.

Case with Error

A 32-year-old woman develops TTP. She is being effectively
treated with apheresis, and her platelet count is below normal
at 35 000 per microliter but rising slightly with each apheresis
procedure. A doctor suggests platelet transfusions for this patient
to raise the platelet count more quickly toward normal. The patient
shows no evidence of neurologic signs and has not experienced a
severe hemorrhage.

Explanation and Consequences

In patients with TTP, platelets could be considered for transfusion
if the thrombocytopenia is so severe that major bleeding is a high
likelihood. However, platelet transfusions in such patients have
been associated with ischemia in the central nervous system and
in other organs. For this reason, in the case described above, platelet transfusions are not indicated despite the presence of significant
thrombocytopenia.

OTHER MISTAKES

▶ The failure of the laboratory to recognize platelet clumps, or clots containing platelets, in the collection tube as a result of inadequate sample mixing with the anticoagulant in the tube at the time of collection, when it is possible to do so. In many cases, the platelet clumps are too small to be recognized visually by the technologist in the laboratory. Platelet clumping in the collection tube can significantly lower than the platelet count when it is quantitated in a cell counter. In such cases, it may be difficult for a treating physician to know that a low platelet count is artifactual and that it is decreased as a result of inadequate mixing of blood and anticoagulant by the person collecting the blood sample. Comparing platelet counts over time, if they are available, can raise the suspicion that a single low platelet count is spurious and not reflective of the patient's true condition.

Case with Error

An inexperienced phlebotomist collects blood samples for complete blood counts and coagulation tests during her first week of employment, but consistently fails to invert the tubes to mix the anticoagulant with the blood immediately after blood collection. Technologists in the clinical laboratory notice that there has been a noticeable increase in the number of samples with visibly apparent platelet clumps and blood clots.

Explanation and Consequences

The error in this case is associated with the poor technique of the phlebotomist. Dried anticoagulants in particular, such as EDTA in purple top vacuum tubes, do not effectively mix with the collected blood unless the tube is gently inverted.

> ▶ Mistaking particulate matter or microorganisms for platelets in a blood sample analyzed in an automated blood cell counter. In some cases, a presumably high platelet count can be further evaluated immediately in the laboratory by review of the raw data from the cell counter to show that particles or microorganisms roughly the same size and density of platelets are being mistaken as platelets. In other cases, however, when it is impossible for the laboratory to convincingly demonstrate that an artifactually high platelet count is spurious, the physician needs to be suspicious that an elevated platelet count is not truly present.

Case with Error

A patient with severe sepsis from Candida is evaluated with the complete blood count. The platelet count is noted to be extremely elevated. Repeat testing for the platelet count shows a persistent elevation while the patient is septic. No explanation for the apparent thrombocytosis is ever established by the doctor.

Explanation and Consequences

On some automated cell counters, organisms such as Candida can masquerade as platelets, and thereby elevate the "platelet count," which is provided by the cell counter. This is not the case for all cell counters, as some are more effective than others at identifying the differences between platelets and microorganisms of a similar size.

STANDARDS OF CARE

▦ The platelet count should be monitored in patients being treated with medications that can lead to thrombocytopenia. The prototype drug in this category is heparin, but other pharmaceutical compounds can also lead to drug-induced thrombocytopenia.

▦ Platelet clumping induced by EDTA in a purple top collection tube containing EDTA as an anticoagulant should be an early consideration in a patient with a low platelet count and no other obvious explanation.

▦ Extremely low platelet counts, especially those below 10 000 per microliter, represent critical values and require immediate attention.

▦ TTP should be considered as a possible diagnosis when thrombocytopenia and the appropriate constellation of clinical and laboratory parameters are present. Prompt institution of apheresis for cases with a high likelihood for TTP is essential.

▦ Platelet concentrates are not indicated as a treatment for thrombocytopenia from all causes. In fact, platelet concentrates may be contraindicated for certain causes of thrombocytopenia, such as HIT.

▦ The laboratory should attempt to recognize platelet clumps in the collection tube as a result of inadequate sample mixing with the anticoagulant in the tube at the time of collection, realizing that this is possible only if the clumps are large.

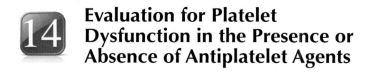

Evaluation for Platelet Dysfunction in the Presence or Absence of Antiplatelet Agents

OVERVIEW

Assessment of platelet function in clinical laboratories has been performed for many decades using platelet-rich plasma and an assortment of platelet agonists, including collagen, arachidonate, ADP, epinephrine, and ristocetin. Performance of this test is associated with many potential analytical errors that must be avoided to provide the most interpretable result for platelet function. Platelet function can also be assessed using whole blood, with the determination of both platelet aggregation and platelet granule release. Markedly abnormal responses to multiple agonists are likely to indicate abnormal platelet function in vivo. However, predictability of bleeding risk in a patient with minor reductions in platelet activity, particularly with a weak platelet agonist like epinephrine, is highly uncertain.

Recently, new assays have been introduced to offer an assessment of platelets for aspirin and clopidogrel (Plavix) resistance. Platelet function can now be evaluated using several different methodologies. Platelet aggregation is now performed not only to assess baseline platelet function but also to determine if an antiplatelet medication has produced the desired platelet inhibition. In this situation, a desired response is often poor platelet function because it implies that the anti-platelet medication is effective.

TEST ORDERING MISTAKES

Performing tests for platelet function, when the patient has purposely or inadvertently ingested aspirin or other anti-platelet medication before testing. Aspirin is included in a number of over-the-counter preparations that do not have the word aspirin in the name. In addition, a number of aspirin preparations have names that do not suggest that the pill or capsule is indeed aspirin. Because of this, patients inadvertently can ingest aspirin and report no aspirin ingestion. In this situation, platelet dysfunction will be observed as a result of the antiplatelet medication and obscure any endogenous abnormalities that might be present and detectable. If aspirin has been avoided for 5 to 7 days, most of the decreased platelet function should be restored. If aspirin has been avoided for 10 to 14 days, in the absence of other variables, platelet function should be fully restored. Recent ingestion of clopidogrel will also result in abnormal platelet function if the patient effectively converts the oral prodrug into the active antiplatelet medication. Platelet function returns to normal approximately 7 days after the last dose of clopidogrel.

Case with Error

A patient is asked to refrain from aspirin before an evaluation for platelet function by platelet aggregation using platelet-rich plasma. The assay is performed, and the result shows no response of the patient's platelets to arachidonate and first-wave platelet aggregation responses only to epinephrine and to ADP. When the patient is questioned about aspirin ingestion that could be present in over-the-counter preparations, she reports that she has taken Alka-Seltzer within the past 24 hours.

Explanation and Consequences

The error in this case is on the part of the patient and is inadvertent. Many preparations contain aspirin, and patients can unknowingly ingest aspirin even when they are attempting to avoid it. This error necessitated repeat performance of a complex assay.

> ▶️ Use of the template bleeding time to assess platelet function. This test is associated with many variables, and currently, it is rarely used to assess the adequacy of platelet function. In particular, it has been shown to be a poorly predictive test for platelet function in the patient anticipating surgery.

Case with Error

A patient is evaluated preoperatively with a bleeding time test. The patient has a negative history for bleeding. The result for the test is prolonged, and the surgery is postponed until a more extensive evaluation for platelet function is performed.

Explanation and Consequences

Although this is uncommon today, the situation occurred many times when the bleeding time test was considered a necessary part of a pre-operative evaluation to fully assess a patient's capacity for hemostasis perioperatively. The error is particularly costly, and the delay in the performance of surgery may be clinically detrimental.

RESULT INTERPRETATION MISTAKES

> Concluding that any reduction in platelet function is associated with an increased risk for bleeding. In a standard platelet-rich plasma–based platelet aggregation study, for example, the clinical significance of a mildly decreased response to epinephrine is highly uncertain. Minor abnormalities may or may not be associated with an increased risk for bleeding.

Case with Error

A patient is evaluated with platelet aggregation studies and is found to have only a mildly decreased response to epinephrine. A diagnosis of a qualitative platelet disorder with a predisposition to bleeding is made, and the doctor notes that before any surgical procedures in the future, this patient will require platelet transfusions.

Explanation and Consequences

The doctor has made definitive conclusions about the patient's ability to aggregate platelets with only a weak indication that the platelets are dysfunctional. Repeat testing at some point is likely to be informative and may show no evidence of impaired aggregation to epinephrine.

> Failing to consider the potential antiplatelet effect of medications taken by a patient being evaluated for platelet function. A careful review of the adverse effect of many pharmaceutical compounds, as well as herbal medicines, indicates that an impairment in platelet function can occur in some percentage of patients taking these drugs. If possible, repeat testing for platelet function in the absence of a drug suspected to be responsible for platelet dysfunction is likely to be informative.

Case with Error

A patient taking large amounts of garlic supplements daily over the past few months experiences a recent onset of easy bruising and is evaluated with platelet aggregation studies. The platelet response to the weaker agonists is impaired. There is a clear temporal association between the initiation of garlic intake at high doses and the development of the easy bruising. The doctor overlooks over-the-counter preparations as potential explanations of impaired platelet aggregation.

Explanation and Consequences

A number of herbal medicines, garlic being one, can impair platelet function in some patients, usually without significant harm to the patient. However, if the patient is predisposed to bleed, by undergoing surgery, for example, the modest platelet function impairment induced by an herbal medication may become clinically important.

OTHER MISTAKES

▶ The failure of the laboratory to appropriately perform the test for platelet aggregation using platelet-rich plasma. Technical variables that can produce false results (positive or negative) include the following: allowing the sample of platelet-rich plasma to sit too long before a platelet agonist is added; cooling the platelet-rich plasma before the addition of the platelet agonist; addition of the platelet agonist to the wall of the tube containing platelet-rich plasma in such a way that the agonist never fully mixes with the platelet suspension; contamination of the platelet-rich plasma with red blood cells that do not clump in the presence of the platelet agonist and obscure the platelet response; and not assessing the activity of platelet agonists with normal donor platelets as controls when the platelet aggregation responses of the patient are reduced.

Case with Error

A blood sample is collected from a patient for platelet aggregation studies. The sample is centrifuged appropriately, and platelet-rich plasma is obtained. The technologist is distracted by another task in the laboratory, and the platelet-rich plasma remains on the laboratory bench before analysis for 2 hours. The platelet aggregation study is then initiated with the addition of platelet agonists. The aggregation response to all of the agonists is markedly impaired. However, the agonists are shown to be active when a control blood sample is collected, appropriately processed to provide platelet-rich plasma, and the agonists added shortly after the normal donor platelet-rich plasma is available.

Explanation and Consequences

The error in this case is allowing the patient's platelet-rich plasma to sit too long before the addition of platelet agonists. After platelets have been removed from the circulation, their function can be assessed for only a short time. Ideally, agonists are added to platelet-rich plasma approximately 30 minutes after the sample has been collected.

CONTROVERSY

There is growing evidence to support the use of pharmacogenomic testing for CYP2C19. This cytochrome system metabolizes clopidogrel from an oral prodrug to an active platelet antagonist. Patients with decreased function of CYP2C19 are poor responders to clopidogrel and suffer an increased frequency of thrombotic events.

A particularly significant controversy relates to the concept of aspirin sensitivity testing. There are several diagnostic platforms in use to assess the sensitivity of platelets to aspirin. The lack of a consensus-driven guideline for aspirin resistance testing is explained by several factors. One is that a single sample of platelets tested on the multiple available diagnostic platforms for aspirin sensitivity is likely to produce mixed results, with some assays suggesting that a patient's platelets are aspirin sensitive and other assays suggesting that the platelets are aspirin resistant. It is impossible to know which test result reflects the true response of the platelets to aspirin in vivo. A second factor is that there is no universally accepted definition of aspirin resistance. A third issue is that apparent aspirin resistance in many patients taking 81 mg of aspirin daily is overcome by simply increasing the dose to 325 mg daily. These patients appear to be aspirin resistant only at a lower aspirin dose. There is one circumstance that has been widely accepted to produce aspirin resistance. It has been shown that ingestion of a nonsteroidal anti-inflammatory drug, such as ibuprofen, shortly preceding aspirin ingestion can prevent the permanent antiplatelet effect induced by aspirin. Platelets can recover adequate function after exposure to a nonsteroidal anti-inflammatory drug, usually within 24 hours after the drug has been taken. Therefore, aspirin-treated platelets that have been previously exposed to a nonsteroidal anti-inflammatory drug are commonly found to be aspirin resistant because they recover platelet function after exposure to aspirin.

STANDARDS OF CARE

▦ When performing a test for platelet function to assess bleeding risk in the absence of antiplatelet medications, it is necessary for the patient to have avoided aspirin and clopidogrel for, ideally, at least 7 to 10 days before testing. Non-steroidal anti-inflammatory drugs (NSAIDs) should be avoided for at least 24 hours.

▦ It is necessary to take a complete history of prescription and nonprescription medications before platelet function testing, to accurately determine if any platelet function defect is a result of inadvertent ingestion of an antiplatelet medication, most commonly aspirin.

▦ Use of the template bleeding time to assess platelet function has been widely abandoned and should not be used to evaluate bleeding risk.

▦ A mild reduction in platelet aggregation, as an isolated laboratory finding, should not be considered as a definite risk factor for bleeding.

▦ The potential antiplatelet effect of all medications, not just known antiplatelet drugs being taken by a patient who is evaluated for platelet function, must always be considered in the interpretation of platelet function tests.

▦ The clinical laboratory must meticulously perform the test for platelet aggregation using platelet-rich plasma to avoid introducing technical variables that can produce false results.

Annotated Bibliography

The following annotated references may be useful in identifying the primary literature for information connected to the standards of care in this textbook.

Colman RW, Hirsh J, Marder VJ, Clowes AW, George JN, eds. Hemostasis and Thrombosis, Basic Principles and Clinical Practice. 5th ed. Philadelphia, PA: Lippincott Williams & Wilkins; 2007.

> *This textbook is encyclopedic in nature with detailed descriptions about the basic and clinical aspects of hemostasis and thrombosis. The list of primary references in each area is very extensive.*

Hillyer CD, Shaz BH, Zimring JC, eds. Part II: Coagulation. In: Transfusion Medicine and Hemostasis: Clinical and Laboratory Aspects. Oxford, UK: Elsevier; 2009:433–750.

> *This textbook covers a wide variety of topics in coagulation. There are selected references for each topic. There is also information that is relevant to the topics in this book that overlap both coagulation and transfusion medicine.*

Marques MB, Fritsma GA. Coagulation Testing. 2nd ed. Washington, DC: AACC Press; 2009.

> *This is a small handbook with practical information. It contains a number of relevant primary references to the diagnosis and treatment of coagulation disorders.*

Michelson AD, ed. Platelets. 2nd ed. Oxford, UK: Academic Press; 2007.

> *This textbook in its second edition has become a major reference for clinical and basic topics related to platelets. This textbook contains detailed reference lists for every topic.*

Van Cott EM, Laposata M. Coagulation. In: Jacobs DS, DeMott WR, Oxley DK, eds. Jacobs and DeMott Laboratory Test Handbook with Key Word Index. 5th ed. Hudson, OH: Lexi-Comp; 2001:327–358.

> *This textbook describes individual laboratory tests. This citation refers to the chapter on coagulation tests. The references are included as footnotes. The focus of each section within the chapter is an individual coagulation laboratory test. The description for each test is provided in significant detail.*

Van Cott EM, Laposata M. Bleeding and thrombotic disorders. In: Laposata M, ed. Laboratory Medicine: The Diagnosis of Disease in the Clinical Laboratory. New York, NY: McGraw-Hill; 2010:chap 11, 235–270.

This book covers the entire field of laboratory medicine. The chapter on bleeding and thrombotic disorders contains brief descriptions of many disorders, and the associated tables in the chapter describe the diagnostic tests useful in making the clinical diagnosis.

Index

DATE DUE

Demco, Inc. 38-293